Shielding Techniques for Radiation Oncology Facilities

Shielding Techniques for Radiation Oncology Facilities

By Patton H. McGinley, Ph.D., D.A.B.R., D.A.B.H.P.

Medical Physics Publishing
Madison, Wisconsin

ISBN: 0-944838-81-2 Hardcover 0-944838-82-0 Softcover

Library of Congress Cataloging-in-Publication Data
McGinley, Patton H., 1935–
Shielding techniques for radiation oncology facilities / by Patton H. McGinley.
p. cm.
Includes bibliographical references and index.
ISBN 0-944838-81-2 (hardcover). -- ISBN 0-944838-82-0 (softcover)
1. Radiology, Medical--Equipment and supplies--Safety measures.
2. Hospitals--Radiological services--Shielding (Radiation)
3. Cancer--Radiotherapy--Safety measures. I. Title.
[DNLM: 1. Radiation Protection--methods. 2. Radiation Oncology--organization & administration. WN 650 M477s 1998]
R920.M34 1988
616.07'57'0289--dc21
DNLM/DLC
for Library of Congress 97-36743
CIP

Medical Physics Publishing
4513 Vernon Blvd.
Madison, WI 53705
(608) 262-4021

Printed in the United States of America.

Contents

7 Special Topics 93

8 Simulator, HDR, and Brachytherapy Rooms 109

9 Reports and Room Surveys 123

References 137

Index 143

Preface

This book is intended to provide an update of shielding methods for radiation-producing devices found in a modern radiation oncology department. The present methods used for medical shielding are based on several National Council on Radiation Protection and Measurements (NCRP) Reports that were issued more than 20 years ago. During this period there have been many changes in the radiation sources and techniques used for radiation therapy that affect shielding techniques. In particular, the use of higher energy dual mode accelerators and high-dose-rate units, the incorporation of various metals in the shield barriers, and changes of the workload of the accelerators due to the use of new modalities for radiation treatment have introduced design problems that are not addressed in the NCRP reports.

This book was developed from a course in shielding that the author initiated several years ago at Emory University. Practical applications and physical understanding are emphasized as opposed to a formal mathematical development of radiation shielding, and the author has endeavored to produce a text with all traces of lecture notes removed. The book can be used as a text for senior or graduate level medical physics courses or health physics courses, or as a reference. It has been assumed that the reader has a background in radiation physics and is familiar with the radiation-producing devices used in radiation oncology. A large number of worked examples and homework problems are included in most chapters, and data are presented to allow numerical solutions to the homework sets. The examples and homework problems were taken from the author's collection and have been tested by students over several years.

I wish to acknowledge the help and advice given by Conny Graves, who undertook the task of coordinating and producing the first draft of the manuscript. I am greatly indebted to the many students who reviewed the initial draft of the text and provided a number of useful suggestions for improving the book. Finally, I wish to express my thanks to my wife, Bennie, to whom this book is dedicated.

PATTON H. MCGINLEY

1

History of X-Ray Room Shielding

In November 1895 Roentgen's discovery of x-rays altered the course of medicine. Within a year skin burns and eye irritation were observed, and by 1900 it was generally accepted that exposure to x-rays produced these problems. As a result of the recognition of the deleterious effects produced by x-rays, shielding techniques and devices were developed. The chronological history of x-ray shielding can be divided into the periods discussed below. Each period is based on the x-ray source in use for radiation treatment at this time.

Years of Discovery (1895–1900)

The first x-ray shielded enclosure was devised by Roentgen (Glasser 1934) almost 100 years ago. The enclosure was not for the purpose of radiation protection but simply to create a dark room to prevent fogging the photographic plates and also to observe the fluorescence produced by x-rays. Zinc sheets were used to fabricate the room, and the x-ray tube was located at a distance of 0.13 m outside one of the walls. A 1.0 mm thick aluminum window with a diameter of 0.46 m allowed the x-ray beam to enter the enclosure.

Measurements of the transmission of x-rays through various materials were made by Roentgen and by Tesla (1896), and the degree of x-ray scattering produced by metals was investigated by Tesla at the same time. Elihu Thomson (1898) suggested the use of an aluminum filter to remove the soft x-rays from the beam, and a lead tube housing and collimator were described by Rollins (1898).

Gas Tube Era (1900–1913)

The x-ray tubes used until about 1913 were only partially evacuated, and the residual gas was needed for the device to operate properly. Positive gas ions bombarded the cathode, causing the liberation of electrons. The electrons were then attracted to the anode, where x-rays were produced. The amount of gas remaining in the tube varied with the time of use, which in turn caused the tube characteristics to change.

It was known at the beginning of this period that lead was very effective in stopping the lower energy x-rays produced by the gas tubes. Rollins (1902) proposed that film could be used to survey x-ray units for health protection purposes. He suggested that if a photographic plate was not fogged in several minutes, the radiation field was not harmful. For this work and his invention of many devices to limit the exposure to the patient and the x-ray operator, Rollins should be considered a major pioneer in the field of radiation protection. In 1904 his collected notes were published in a private printing (Rollins 1904).

During the gas tube era more evidence of the ability of x-rays to produce cancer and radiodermatitis was collected, and the basic knowledge for radiological protection was established. However, little was done toward formulating radiation protection techniques.

Golden Age of X-Ray Generators (1913–1940)

In 1903, Coolidge developed the hot cathode tube, which yielded a readily controlled and higher energy x-ray source than the gas tube. The 200 kV Coolidge tube was standard equipment for "deep therapy" during the period 1913 to 1940.

The initial attempt to devise x-ray protection methods was undertaken by the British Roentgen Society in 1915 (Henshaw 1945). Due to the war then raging in Europe, little progress was made. Within a few years the death of a number of early radiation workers prompted public reaction, and the American Roentgen Ray Society organized the first radiation protection committee in September 1920 (Henshaw 1945). The next year the British formed the X-Ray and Radium Protection Committee, and by June 1921 recommendations were reported. By September 1922 the American committee published radiation protection recommendations that were quite similar to those of the British. Both reports emphasized the use of lead to attenuate the x-ray beam and distance to reduce the exposure. It was suggested that the tube should be placed in a metal housing and that lead should be used in the walls of the treatment room to protect the operator. For superficial therapy carried out at or below 100 kV, a tube shield equivalent to 2.0 mm of lead was recommended and the walls and viewing window of the treatment room were to be equivalent to 2.0 mm lead. For x-ray tubes operated above 100 kV, the tube housing, view window, and walls were required to be equivalent to 3.0 mm lead.

A scheme of radiation shielding design that is still in use today was devised by Mutscheller (1925) during this period. The thickness of shielding material required to protect the operator was based on the amount of time per day the x-ray generator was operated, the tube current, and the distance from the x-ray source to the operator. Mutscheller considered the tolerance dose to be .01 of the erythema dose per month, which is approximately 0.06 Gy in a month's time.

The erythema dose per month (E) was calculated without shielding by use of equation 1-1.

$$E = \frac{36.8It}{d^2} \tag{1-1}$$

In equation 1-1, I is the tube current in mA, t is the time of operation per month in min, 36.8 is an empirical factor, and d is the distance from the target to the operator in centimeters. The required shielding thickness is calculated based on the fractional reduction of the beam intensity needed to deliver .01 of the erythema dose in one month. Tables were published by Mutscheller listing the thickness of lead needed to reduce the dose to the protection limit as a function of the tube voltage.

The next year Mutscheller (1926) reported on a method to evaluate the radiation scattered by the patient and the surfaces of the treatment room. The scattered radiation (E_s) is given in terms of the erythema dose by equation 1-2.

$$E_s = \frac{E_p SF(50)^2}{d^2} \tag{1-2}$$

In equation 1-2, E_p is the primary erythema dose delivered to the scattering object, S is the area of the exposed surface in square centimeters, F is a scattering coefficient for the material from which the scatter occurs, and d is the distance from the scattering object to the operator in centimeters. Mutscheller reported values of F for a number of materials, measured at 50 cm from the scattering object and normalized to unit area (cm^2).

The total amount of shielding material needed for protection from scattered and direct radiation was calculated using equations 1-1 and 1-2. Part of the required shielding is used to house the tube and provide patient protection, and the remaining material is placed in the walls of the treatment room. Kaye (1927) suggested that a factor to account for occasional occupancy outside the shielding walls should also be used in shielding design.

The second International Congress of Radiology met in 1928 and formed the International Committee on X-Ray and Radium Protection, which was later named the International Committee on Radiation Protection (ICRP). By July 1928, the International Committee on X-Ray and Radium Protection had issued a set of recommendations on radiation safety. At about the same time the United States formed the Advisory Committee on X-Ray and Radium Protection. A report by the Advisory Committee was issued as U.S. Bureau of Standards Handbook No. 15 in 1931. The only shielding data presented in Handbook No. 15 were included in a table listing the minimum lead thickness needed for protection from x-rays produced at voltages ranging from 75 kV to 600 kV. Protection from direct radiation was to be provided by a tube shield whose thickness was determined from the minimum lead thickness table. The thickness of the tube shield could be reduced by an amount equivalent to the lead shielding in the walls, but in no case should the tube enclosure be less than half the total thickness required.

The concept of a primary barrier was introduced for x-ray beams that were fixed in direction. The primary barrier was considered to be the part of a room surface area that could be struck by the x-ray beam.

It was required that the primary barrier extend 0.304 m outside the maximum beam size, a rule that is still used today. The thickness of the primary barrier was obtained from the table based on the voltage of the x-ray generator, and the portion of the room not intercepted by the x-ray beam (secondary barrier) was to be lined with lead 1.0 mm thinner than the primary barrier. On July 24, 1936, Handbook No. 15 was replaced by Handbook No. 20, which contained only slight changes in the shielding requirements for therapy rooms.

Research was begun before 1930 to increase the operating voltage of the x-ray tubes well above 200 kV in order to treat deep-seated tumors with minimum damage to the intervening healthy tissues. By 1933 several x-ray facilities could produce tube voltage on the order of 1 MV. Air was used as the insulator, and flash over was a common problem. To minimize arcing, the tubes were made as long as nine meters, and a special building was needed to house the x-ray generator and tube. To overcome the insulation problem, resonance transformer units and Van de Graaf generators were mounted in steel tanks filled with insulating gas. Using this technique, voltage of two MV was in use by 1939, but the units were still bulky.

Early Betatrons and Linear Accelerators (1941–1960)

Researchers realized that in order to perform deep therapy with precise control of the beam direction, a smaller, more compact x-ray generator was needed. In order to reduce the size, insulation problems needed to be resolved. The first high-energy medical accelerator that did not rely on the production of extremely high voltages was the betatron developed by Kerst (1941). In this device the electron is accelerated in a circular orbit maintained by the perpendicular field of an AC magnet. With each revolution the electron gains energy as it passes through a small potential difference. When it reaches the desired energy it is extracted from orbit to hit the x-ray target. Medical betatrons operating in the energy range of 15 to 45 MeV were in use for cancer therapy until the early 1980s.

The linear accelerator was also developed during this period, and the first patient was treated at the Hammersmith Hospital in England in 1953. In the linear accelerator the electron is accelerated across a moderate voltage in a repetitive manner along a linear path. Medical linear accelerators operating as high as 25 MeV have replaced the betatron for use in cancer therapy.

The Advisory Committee on X-Ray and Radium Protection was renamed the National Council on Radiation Protection and Measurement (NCRP) in 1946. The NCRP recommended in 1948 that the radiation protection level be reduced from 0.1 R per day to 0.3 R per week. In 1950 the International Commission on Radiation Units and Measurements (ICRU) was formed to replace the International Committee on X-Ray and Radium Protection. As a result of a combined meeting of the NCRP and ICRU in 1953, the permissible dose was lowered to 5 R per year.

For the first time in the National Bureau of Standards (NBS) Handbook No. 60 (NBS 1955), the NCRP suggested the use of the technique proposed by Mutscheller (1925, 1926) for shielding calculations for primary and secondary barriers. Equation 1-3 was used to determine the required transmission factor (K) for primary barriers, and then the shield thickness was read from transmission curves given in the handbook.

$$K = \frac{PD^2}{WUT} \tag{1-3}$$

In equation 1-3 P is the protection dose limit per week, D is the distance (m) from the x-ray target to the point to be protected, and W is the workload at one m from the target in dose per week. The occupancy factor (T) is the fraction of the time that a person is expected to occupy the area outside the barrier, and the use factor (U) is the fraction of the time the x-ray beam falls on the barrier.

Secondary barriers receive only radiation leaking through the tube housing and radiation scattered from materials in the primary beam. The secondary barrier thickness required for 90° scattered radiation is given by equation 1-4.

$$K = \frac{1000PD^2}{WT} \tag{1-4}$$

Now D is the distance from the scattering object to the point protected, and all other symbols have the same meaning as those of equation 1-3. Note that the use factor (U) is always one for secondary radiation. The factor of 1000 appears in equation 1-4 because the ratio of the primary to the scattered radiation at one meter from the object is 1000/1 when the distance from the x-ray target to the scattering object is also one meter. The thickness of the secondary barrier for scattered radiation is now determined from tables of K versus the tube operating voltage given in NBS Handbook No. 60. The barrier thickness based on the leakage radiation is also determined from tables given in the handbook. Since the barrier is subjected to both leakage and scattered radiation, it is now necessary to determine the thickness of shielding that will reduce the sum of radiation components to the protection level. A rule of thumb that is still in use today is if the thickness of the barrier is about the same for each component, one half value layer (HVL) is added to the barrier thickness; if the two thicknesses differ by 3 HVLs or more, the larger barrier thickness is used.

Modern Radiation Therapy Period (1960–Present)

The present methods of calculating the thickness of the primary and secondary barrier for x-rays are fully described in NCRP Report No. 49 (NCRP 1976), Report No. 51 (NCRP 1977), and Report No. 79 (1984). The basic calculation techniques for shielding are similar to those given in NBS Handbook No. 60 except as noted below. Report No. 49 is used for photon energies up to 10 MeV, and Report No. 51 is employed for higher photon energies. Detailed shielding information for neutrons produced by high-energy x-ray interactions is given in NCRP Report No. 79. The design of mazes for photons and neutrons was introduced for the first time in NCRP Report No. 51, and Report No. 79 contains additional information about mazes used to attenuate neutrons.

The present shielding method relies on data, in either tabular or graphical form, in conjunction with simple empirical equations to design shielding for medical facilities. This method of shield design is adequate for high-energy therapy rooms constructed of concrete. However, when the energy of the accelerator exceeds 10 MeV and lead or steel is used to provide part of the shielding, complications are introduced by the generation of neutrons by photon interactions in the shielding and by high-energy photons produced by neutron interactions. Due to the limited data that exist for high-energy medical accelerators the shield designer is forced to rely on past experience.

In July 1995 the NCRP appointed a Scientific Committee to rectify this situation. The committee will prepare an updated report on structural shielding and facility design for medical use of x-rays and gamma rays in the energy range 0.25 to 50 MeV.

2

Conventional Shield Design

Calculation Methods

At present, shielding design for accelerators operating at 10 MeV or less is based on information given in NCRP Report No. 49 (NCRP 1976), and NCRP Report No. 51 (NCRP 1977) is used for higher energy machines. These reports are based on simple empirical equations similar to those developed by Mutscheller (1925 and 1926). Figure 2-1 shows a typical room plan for a high-energy (≥ 15 MeV) medical accelerator. Two types of radiation barriers or shields are considered—primary and secondary. The primary barrier is irradiated by the x-ray beam produced by the accelerator, and the secondary barrier receives only radiation scattered by the patient and the surfaces of the treatment room and radiation transmitted through the accelerator shielding (head leakage). Primary radiation is limited in direction by the placement of the accelerator in the treatment room, and the maximum beam size is used to determine the portion of the walls, ceiling, and floor that will be designated as primary barriers. Secondary radiation, however, is emitted in all directions and covers all of the treatment room surfaces.

The transmission of the barrier (B_x) required to reduce the primary radiation field to an acceptable level outside the barrier is given by

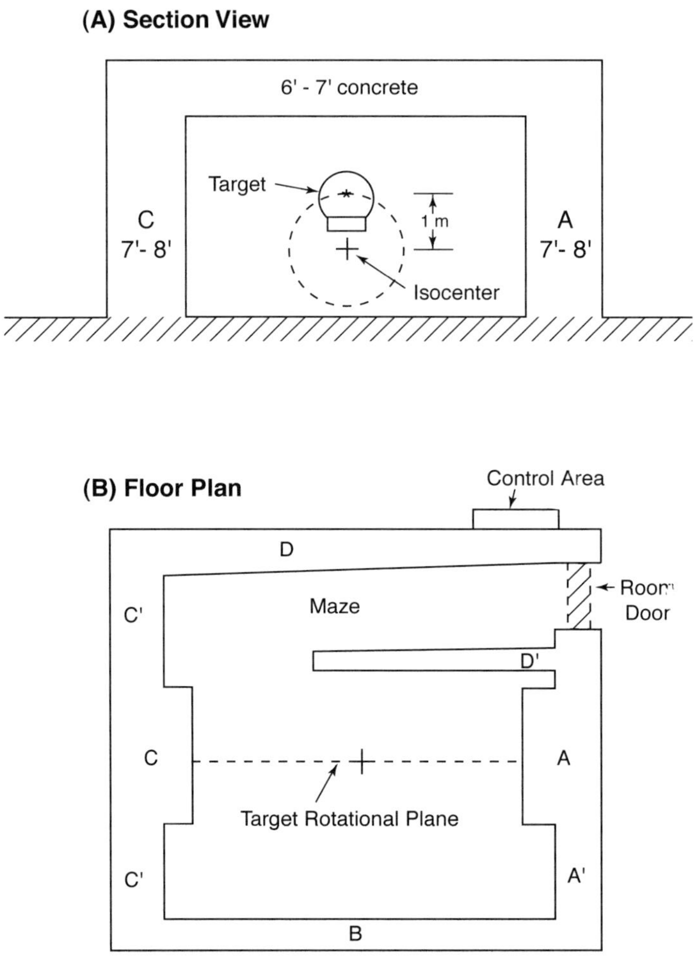

Figure 2-1. Simplified schematic of a typical high-energy treatment room. All barriers are constructed of concrete (147 lb/cubic foot). (A) View in target rotational plane. The path of the target as the gantry rotates is shown by dotted circle. The distance from the isocenter to the floor is 1.3 m. (B) Floor plan view. Secondary walls are A′, B, C′, D, and D′. Each is 3′-4′ thick except D and D′.

equation 2-1. The thickness of the barrier is next determined from curves of B_x versus the shield thickness or calculation using tenth value lengths (TVL) based on the energy of the beam and the type of shielding material.

$$B_x = \frac{P(d_{pri})^2}{WUT} \tag{2-1}$$

In equation 2-1, P is the dose per week required outside the barrier for protection; d_{pri} is the distance from the x-ray target to the point protected in meters; W is the workload, or dose per week at one meter from the target; U is the use factor, or fraction of the time per week that the primary beam falls on the barrier; and T is the occupancy factor, or the fraction of the time that a person will be in the area outside the barrier. The point protected is usually assumed to be 0.305 m outside the radiation barrier in question.

For secondary barriers, the use factor (U) is equal to one, and both the head leakage and scattered radiation shielding requirements must be considered. The barrier transmission needed for radiation scattered from the patient (B_P) is given by equation 2-2.

$$B_p = \frac{P}{aWT} (d_{sec})^2 (d_{sca})^2 \frac{400}{F} \qquad (2\text{-}2)$$

where

d_{sec} = the distance from the scattering surface to the point to be protected (m)

d_{sca} = the distance from the x-ray target to the patient (m)

a = ratio of scattered radiation at one meter from the scattering object to the primary radiation at one meter from the x-ray target

F = beam size at patient (cm^2).

The barrier transmission factor for radiation scattered when the primary beam strikes a barrier is given by equation 2-3.

$$B_s = \frac{P d_{sca}^2 \, d_{sec}^2}{\alpha AWTU} \qquad (2\text{-}3)$$

where

d_{sca} = distance from target to scattering surface (m)

d_{sec} = distance from scattering surface to the point protected (m)

α = reflection coefficient for the barrier material, scattering angle, and x-ray beam energy

A = area of beam at the scattering surface (m^2).

The terms P, W, T, and U in equation 2-3 have been defined above.

The equation shown below can be used to determine the barrier transmission needed for leakage radiation (B_l).

$$B_1 = \frac{1000\ P\ (d_{sec})^2}{WT} \qquad (2\text{-}4)$$

The factor of 1000 appears in equation 2-4 because the head shielding of medical accelerators attenuates the radiation by at least this factor. Since the average position of the x-ray source is the isocenter of the accelerator, the distance d_{sec} is the distance from the isocenter to the point protected. However, a special case for d_{sec} occurs for an accelerator with a horizontal wave guide. For the secondary barrier behind the accelerator, the distance from the gun to the point outside the barrier should be used for d_{sec} because this barrier is subjected primarily to leakage radiation from the vicinity of the gun.

The variables (W, U, T, and P) must now be selected for equations 2-1, 2-2, 2-3, and 2-4 in order to calculate the barrier transmission factor and barrier thickness. The maximum permissible dose equivalent (P) for areas where the general public could be exposed (uncontrolled areas) is set at 1.0 mSv per year. For design purposes a value of 0.02 mSv per week is used in the above equations. In addition, for uncontrolled areas the maximum dose equivalent in any one hour of operation must be 0.02 mSv or less with the occupancy factor equal to one. The value of P required for protection of radiation workers is 0.05 Sv per year. Based on the philosophy of reducing the radiation level to as low as reasonably achievable (ALARA), a shielding design level of 0.10 mSv per week is used for controlled areas where only radiation workers are present. It is also common practice to use a value of one for the occupancy factor (T) for radiation workers. The state radiological health programs have accepted the following conditions as meeting the 1.0 mSv per year and 0.02 mSv in any one hour limits for uncontrolled areas to be satisfied if either of the following conditions is met:

1. If an individual were continually present (T = 1) in an uncontrolled area at the point of maximum exposure, the dose to that individual would not exceed 0.02 mSv in one hour and 0.50 mSv in any year; or

2. If it can be demonstrated by measurement, calculation, or appropriate simulation model that the dose to the individual who is likely to receive the highest dose does not exceed the 1.0 mSv annual dose limit.

Note that method one does not permit the use of occupancy factors other than one and that the annual dose limit has been reduced by a factor of two. The second technique allows the occupancy factor to be less than one, but the shield designer may have to negotiate the value of T with state personnel. The one hour limit of 0.02 mSv does not apply for the second method, and an annual dose equivalent of 1.0 mSv is used.

When selecting the workload (W), one chooses the maximum expected value of the dose at a meter from the target in place of an average value. Most shield designs seem to be based on the value given in NCRP Report No. 49 of 1,000 Gy per week for x-ray beams in the range 0.5 to 10 MV and the value of 500 Gy per week given in NCRP Report No. 51 for higher energy machines. It should be pointed out that these values were established by the NCRP in the mid-1970s before the development of multienergy and multimodality medical accelerators. These workloads were intended for use by "busy departments," where W values were not available.

A recent survey of four modern radiation oncology departments (ten dual energy machines and three single energy machines) by Klech et al. (1994) indicated that the single energy accelerators (6 MV) had a workload less than 350 Gy per week and that the dual energy accelerator workloads were less than 250 Gy per week for the high-energy x-ray beam. Note that the shielding requirements for dual energy accelerators are dominated by the high-energy x-ray beam and that the workload for the 6 MV beam has only a moderate influence on the shielding design. The workload for the electron beam can be disregarded due to the limited penetration of electrons. When determining that the shielding is adequate to prevent the dose equivalent from exceeding 0.02 mSv in any one hour of operation for uncontrolled areas, a workload of 20 Gy at one meter from the target in one hour is a reasonable value to assume. To be conservative, both the use factor (U) and occupancy factor (T) are made equal to one.

If total body photon treatment is to be conducted with the accelerator, a major adjustment of the workload will be needed and one of the primary wall barriers will have to be increased in thickness (Barish 1996). When total body photon therapy is carried out, the patient is positioned near one of the primary walls in order to secure a field size large enough to encompass the whole patient. To deliver an adequate x-ray dose to the patient, the dose at the isocenter must become large. For example, if a total body dose of 14 Gy is given at a depth of 10 cm in a patient positioned at 3.67 m from the x-ray target, approximately 241 Gy dose will be delivered at the isocenter for a 6 MV x-ray beam. The treatment is carried out over a time interval of less than one week, thereby increasing the weekly and hourly workload.

Use factors of 25% for each wall, ceiling, and floor were recommended by the NCRP in the 1970s. These values are now commonly used by shield designers. It should be pointed out that for total body photon therapy one primary wall will have a relatively large use factor due to the high dose level required at the isocenter.

The scatter-primary ratio (a) in equation 2-2 changes with the scattering angle and the energy of the accelerator. NCRP Report No. 49 contains limited data for the scatter of medical linac beams by the patient, listing only one value for a 4 MV beam (a=0.0027 for 45° scatter). Table 2-1 lists the scatter-primary ratio given for 6 MV and10 MV.

Table 2-1 Scatter-primary ratio (a) at one meter from a human-size phantom for a size 400 cm^2 at the phantom, target to phantom distance of one meter

Scattering angle (deg)	*6 MV** *a*	*10 MV*† *a*
30	0.007	0.0030
45	0.0018	0.0010
60	0.0011	0.0005
90	0.0006	0.0003
135	0.0004	0.0002

*From NCRP Report No. 49.

†From Weise and Jost (1983).

Values of the reflection coefficient α can be obtained from Figure 3-3, which was reproduced from NCRP Report No. 51 (NCRP 1977). Since scattered radiation has rather low penetration compared with head leakage and primary beam radiation for accelerators operating above 10 MV, it can be ignored for barrier calculations.

Occupancy factors (T) have been suggested by the NCRP (NCRP 1976) for the case where values are not available; these are presented in Table 2-2.

Table 2-2 Occupancy factors (T) for nonoccupationally exposed personnel*

T	Type of area
1	Full Occupancy: work areas such as offices, shops, laboratories, children's play areas, occupied nearby buildings, living quarters, wards, nurses' stations
1/4	Partial Occupancy: corridors, rest rooms, elevators using operators [I have not seen one of these in years], unattended parking lots
1/16	Occasional Occupancy: waiting rooms, toilets, stairways, unattended elevators, janitors' closets, outside areas used only for pedestrians or vehicular traffic

*From NCRP Report No. 49 (NCRP 1976).

The values shown in Table 2-2 can be used in calculating the barrier transmission factor required to reduce the exposure from the source to 0.02 mSv per week or 1.0 mSv per year in uncontrolled areas, but a T value of one is used to evaluate the barrier transmission needed to ensure that nonoccupational personnel are not exposed to more than 0.02 mSv in any one hour of operation.

Barrier Materials

Table 2-3 summarizes the physical properties of common shielding materials. Concrete has the advantage of low cost, but its relatively low density and average atomic number may require considerable thickness. Concrete is usually poured into a form that contains reinforcing rods that provide tensile strength. When possible, the pour should be continuous in order to eliminate seams. Voids are prevented by having the concrete sufficiently fluid when it is cast. Heavy or high-density concrete can be used to reduce the shield thickness when space is limited, but the cost per unit mass is greater than for ordinary concrete. Concrete should not be heated above 93° C due to the rapid loss of water. The thicknesses of concrete shields are normally based on ordinary concrete, which has a density of 2.35 g cm^{-3} (147 lb ft^{-3}). It is therefore common practice to determine the density of the concrete when it is poured. An adjustment can be made in the thickness of the shield based on the ratio of the measured density to the density of ordinary concrete. Numark and Kase (1985) have pointed out that the wall thickness required for normal concrete should not be converted to the equivalent thickness of heavy concrete by use of the density ratio. If one uses the density ratio, an overestimation of the heavy concrete shield thickness on the order of a factor of two to four will result. The overestimation of concrete thickness was attributed to the higher average atomic number of the heavy concrete as compared with ordinary concrete. Numark and Kase (1985) recommend that measured transmission data for heavy concrete (Lokan et al. 1972 and Maruyama et al. 1971) be used for the design of shields.

The properties of low-carbon steel or iron are given in Table 2-3. These materials have a medium density and atomic number and are less expensive per unit mass than lead. Steel has high strength relative to lead, and it can be used as a structural component. For example, door frames and cases for high-energy accelerator rooms are usually fabricated of 0.6 cm thick steel.

If a shield of minimum thickness is required, lead can be used. However, lead sheets tend to flow due to their weight and must be supported by attaching the sheet to a concrete wall or ceiling or by laminating the lead in structural materials, such as concrete or steel. When lead is attached to a concrete wall or ceiling with steel studs, a leakage path for x-rays is created due to the lower density and atomic number of the steel. In particular, a stud located at a point in a barrier intercepted by the beam may cause excessive radiation leakage, and additional shielding may need to be added. Lead has the additional disadvantage of high cost and low strength. Earth is an inexpensive shielding material, and it can be used to fill the region between two concrete retaining walls. The x-ray attenuation offered by earth depends on the density and composition, both of which are quite variable.

Table 2-3 Physical properties of common shielding materials*

Shielding material	*Density ($g\text{-}cm^3$)*	*Atomic number*	*Relative cost per unit mass*†	*Tensile strength (psi)*
ordinary concrete	2.3	11	1.0	500
heavy concrete	3.7–4.8	26	5.8	—
low-carbon steel	7.87	26	2.2	40,000
lead	11.35	82	22.2	1,900
earth, dry packed	1.5	—	low	—

*Data for concrete, steel, and lead from Profio (1979) and earth from NCRP (1977).

†Relative cost normalized to a cost of one for ordinary concrete.

Barrier Thickness

Once the barrier transmission factor has been calculated, the thickness of the required shielding material can be determined based on broad beam transmission data. NCRP Reports No. 49 and No. 51 are convenient sources of graphical data for primary and secondary barriers composed of concrete, steel, and lead. However, the curves are limited to a few megavoltages and modest thicknesses of shielding materials. With knowledge of the barrier transmission factor, the barrier thickness can be read directly from the appropriate graph. When data are not available for leakage radiation, it is recommended that the primary curve for 60% of the nominal accelerating potential be used. A second approach based on TVLs is given in NCRP Report No. 51. Both the first TVL (T_1) and equilibrium, or subsequent, TVL (T_e) are given in NCRP Report No. 51 for lead, concrete, and steel. Table 2-4 is a summary of the NCRP values for TVLs.

Table 2-4 Tenth value layers in ordinary concrete, steel, and lead*

Electron energy (MeV)	*Shield material*	*TVL_1 (m)*	*TVL_e (m)*
6	concrete	0.35	0.35
	steel	0.099	0.099
	lead	0.055	0.057
10	concrete	0.41	0.39
	steel	0.104	0.104
	lead	0.057	0.056
15	concrete	0.46	0.43
	steel	0.108	0.108
18	concrete	0.47	0.43
	steel	0.108	0.108
20	concrete	0.48	0.44
	steel	0.108	0.109
24	concrete	0.51	0.46
	steel	0.109	0.109

*Adapted from figures E.12, E.13, and E.14 of NCRP Report No. 51 (NCRP 1977).

The number (n) of TVLs required for the shield can be obtained from equation 2-5 using the value of the barrier transmission factor (B_x).

$$n = \log_{10}(1/B_x) \tag{2-5}$$

The thickness (S) of the shield is then given by equation 2-6.

$$S = T_1 + (n-1)T_e \tag{2-6}$$

Information that can be used to evaluate the secondary barrier thickness is not given in NCRP Report No. 51. However, for accelerators operating above 10 MV, the scattered radiation component of the secondary radiation is negligible as compared with the head leakage. To be conservative the secondary shield thickness can be calculated using the primary beam TVL. This procedure will result in the secondary barrier being overshielded.

Varian Corporation, a major manufacturer of medical linear accelerators, provides TVL data for primary beam and 90° head leakage radiation (Varian 1991). A single TVL value, which appears to be based on the average value of the first and third TVL, is used for barrier thickness determination. The average TVL values were obtained from the data given by Nelson and LaRiviere (1984). The TVL values apply for concrete, steel, lead, and earth and are tabulated based on the megavoltage of the accelerator as shown in Table 2-5. One should be careful using this data because the megavoltage is based on information given in the British Journal of Radiology Supplement No. 11 (BJR 1972); other methods of specifying the megavoltage are in common use and give different values of the megavoltage. For comparison, Table 2-6 gives megavoltage values based on the British Journal of Radiology Supplements No. 11 (BJR 1972) and No. 17 (BJR 1983).

Nelson and LaRiviere (1984) have also published TVL information for head leakage radiation emitted at angles from 35 to 145° to the target. Table 2-7 lists the TVL values for head leakage penetration in ordinary concrete.

If the radiation is obliquely incident on the shielding barrier as shown in figure 2-2, the barrier thickness can be reduced. A "rule of thumb" for the required thickness based on cobalt-60 and cesium-137 gamma radiation is presented in NCRP Report No. 49. The radiation path length (t) is given by

$$t = S/\cos\Theta \tag{2-7}$$

where S is the thickness of the barrier and θ is the angle of the beam with respect to the normal to the barrier. The rule of thumb is outlined below.

Table 2-5 Tenth value layers for primary and secondary leakage radiation at 90° *

X-ray megavoltage†	*Shielding material*	*TVL primary (m)*	*TVL 90° leakage (m)*
6	concrete	0.343	0.279
	earth	0.572	—
	steel	0.098	0.080
	lead	0.055	0.045
10	concrete	0.389	0.305
	earth	0.648	—
	steel	0.105	0.085
	lead	0.056	0.046
15	concrete	0.432	0.330
	earth	0.720	—
	steel	0.108	0.087
	lead	0.057	0.047
18	concrete	0.444	0.330
	earth	0.740	—
	steel	0.111	0.087
	lead	0.056	0.047
20	concrete	0.457	0.343
	steel	0.112	0.088
	lead	0.055	0.049
24	concrete	0.470	0.356
	steel	0.107	0.089
	lead	0.052	0.051

*Adapted from Varian (1991).

†Megavoltage based on values from the British Journal of Radiology Suppl. 11 (1972).

Table 2-6 BJR Supplements No. 11 and No. 17 corresponding megavoltage values

BJR #11	4	6	10	15	18	20	24 MV
BJR #17	4	6	10	16	23	25	30 MV

Table 2-7 First and third TVLs for head leakage radiation*

Electron energy (MeV)	*6*	*10*	*25*
Angle	*TVL_1/TVL_3 (m)*	*TVL_1/TVL_3 (m)*	*TVL_1/TVL_3 (m)*
35°–55°	0.353/0.293	0.366/0.328	0.377/0.367
80°–100°	0.341/0.284	0.349/0.311	0.359/0.347
125°–145°	0.333/0.269	0.347/0.299	0.355/0.325

*Adapted from Nelson and LaRiviere (1984) for ordinary concrete.

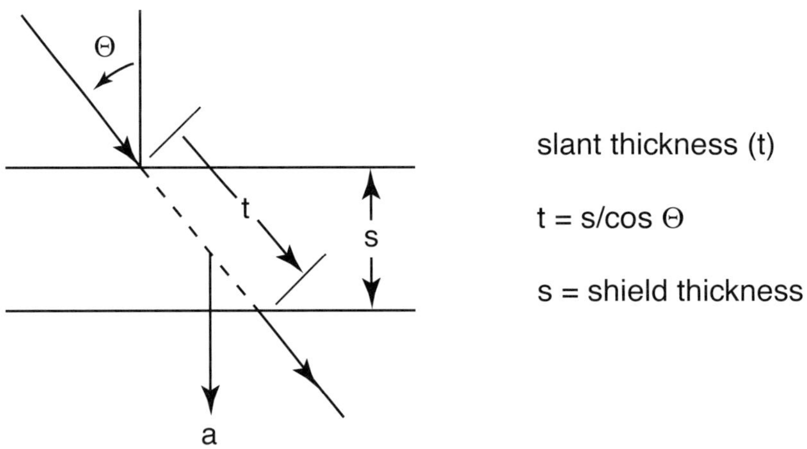

Figure 2-2. Oblique incident radiation beam and slant thickness (t)

1. If the barrier is composed of concrete, an attenuation of 1000 is required, and θ is 50°, increase the barrier two HVLs for low-energy radiation and one HVL for high-energy radiation. The additional shielding is needed to account for scattered radiation, as shown by ray (a) in figure 2-2.
2. For angles of 60° and 70° each of the above thicknesses need to be increased by one and two HVLs respectively.
3. For lead shields with a required attenuation of 1000, the barrier is increased by one HVL at 60°.

4. The minimum angle of obliquity is used to evaluate the attenuation for a diverging beam.

These rules are commonly used in the design of shields for high-energy x-rays even though the validity of the rules has only recently been investigated. Biggs (1996), using data for beams of cobalt-60, 4, 10, and 18 MV x-rays, tested the use of obliquity rules and found the following for values of θ in the range from 0° to 70°.

1. For cobalt-60 and $\theta < 45°$, deviations from obliquity are noticeable for barrier transmission factors less than 4×10^{-3}; for $\theta = 60°$, they are noticeable below 1×10^{-2}.
2. The concrete shielding thickness for x-rays of 10 MV or greater can be based on the slant thickness (t) providing θ is less than 70°.
3. For steel the slant thickness should not be used for an 18 MV beam if the value of θ is greater than 60° and t is greater than 35 cm.
4. For lead the slant thickness should not be used for an 18 MV beam if the value of θ is greater than 60° and t is greater than 17 cm.

The reader is referred to Biggs's publication for detailed information about the slant thickness needed for high-energy x-rays.

Width and Length of Primary Barrier

As mentioned in chapter 1, the primary barrier width is made equivalent to the maximum beam size at the barrier plus one foot (0.305 m) on either side to prevent radiation from leaking through the secondary barrier that abuts the primary. The maximum beam size for most accelerators at one meter from the target is 40×40 cm². However, by rotating the collimator 45° from the zero position, the maximum horizon width of the beam is the diagonal dimension of the 40×40 cm² beam (56.6 cm). If the beam is projected on a barrier X meters away, the maximum beam width at the barrier (W′) is given by equation 2-8.

$$W' = 0.566X \tag{2-8}$$

The required horizontal barrier width (W) in meters is given by equation 2-9.

$$W = 0.566X + 0.61 \tag{2-9}$$

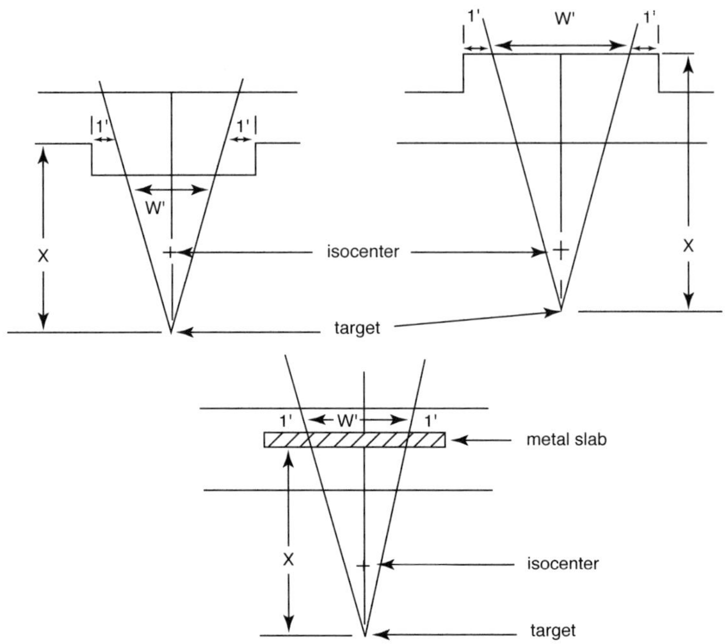

Figure 2-3. Width of primary barriers

Figure 2-3 shows several possible arrangements of the shield and W. For a room fabricated entirely of concrete it is common practice to determine W′ for situations in which the beam is aimed at the junction between the wall and ceiling. This gives the maximum value of W′ for any gantry angle. The wall and ceiling barriers are then constructed with a uniform width of W′ plus 0.61 m. If the ceiling primary is a combination of concrete and metal slabs, the metal portion is tapered to reduce the cost and weight. Figure 2-4 shows views depicting the placement of the metal slab on the concrete barrier. The metal slab immediately above the isocenter has equal length and width ($W_1 = L_1$), and the size in meters is given by equation 2-10 with i equal to one.

$$W_i = 0.566X_{i+1} + 0.61 \qquad (2\text{-}10)$$

In equation 2-10, i is the slab index and the center section has an i value of 1. The distance X_{i+1} is the distance from the x-ray target to the metal slab, as shown in figure 2-4. The remainder of the metal portion of the ceiling barrier is made up of a series of sections of increasing width but equal length (L). Typically L has a value of about 1.8 m for each section. However, the last section (maximum i) may be more

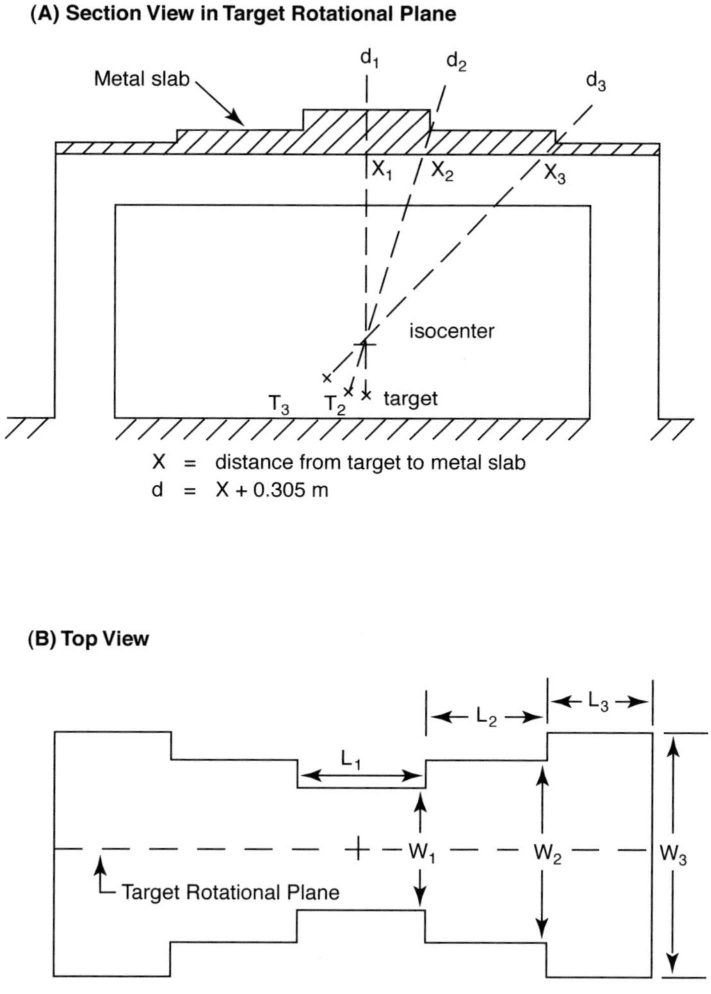

Figure 2-4. Tapered metal slab for ceiling primary barrier

or less than L in order to cover the complete length of the room. Note that the barrier transmission factor changes with gantry angle, since d_i increases when the beam is directed toward the ceiling but not vertically up. In addition, the use factor (U_i) for these gantry angles is less than one—on the order of 1/10 or less. The changes in d_i and U_i both increase the barrier transmission factor, which leads to a reduction of the shielding thickness.

One design for the ceiling primary barrier uses at least one foot of concrete for structural strength with the metal slab on top of the concrete. Since it is desirable to reduce the weight and cost of the shield, the metal portion is tapered. It is impractical to taper the concrete part of the ceiling slab due to the extra cost of forms. For accelerators operating above 10 MeV it may be necessary to place neutron shielding on top of the metal layer to protect against photoneutrons produced when the beam strikes the metal part of the ceiling shield. The topic of neutron shielding is covered in chapter 6.

Example Calculations

1. Evaluate the thickness of concrete needed for the primary shield shown below. The beam is 20 MV, and the workload (W) is 500 Gy per week at the isocenter. Carry out the evaluation using the following methods:
   a. Curve E.8 from NCRP Report No. 51
   b. First and equilibrium TVL method (see Table 2-4)
   c. Varian TVL data (Table 2-5)

   The barrier transmission factor (B_x) is calculated as shown below.

$$B_x = \frac{(P)(d)^2}{(W)(T)(U)}$$

A protection level of 0.0001 Sv per week is used as the ALARA level for occupationally exposed personnel.

$$B_x = \frac{(0.0001)(4.4)^2}{(500)(1)(1/4)}$$

$$B_x = 1.55 \times 10^{-5}$$

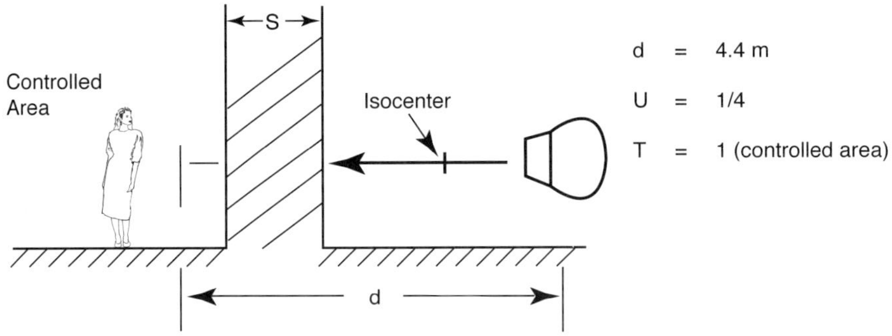

Figure 2-4. Primary barrier for controlled area

a. From NCRP Report No. 51 Curve E.8, for $B = 1.55 \times 10^{-5}$ read $S = 2.21$ m ordinary concrete (147 lb/cubic foot).

b. From Table 2-4, $T_1 = 0.48$ m for a 20 MV x-ray beam and $T_e = 0.44$ m ordinary concrete. The number of TVLs needed is given by:

$$n = \log_{10} (1/B_x) = 4.81 \text{ TVLs}$$

and the thickness (S) is given by:

$$S = T_1 + (n - 1)(T_e) = 0.48 + (4.81 - 1)(0.44)$$

$$S = 2.16 \text{ m ordinary concrete.}$$

c. Varian data (Table 2-5) give 0.457 m TVL for a 20 MV x-ray beam in concrete and

$$S = (n)(TVL) = (4.81)(0.457) = 2.20 \text{ m concrete.}$$

2. Find the width (W) of the primary barrier of example 1c. The primary barrier protrudes into the room, and the adjacent secondary wall is 0.91 m thick. The distance X is given by:

$$X = d - 0.91 - 0.305$$

$$X = 4.4 - 0.91 - 0.305 = 3.2 \text{ m}$$

and the barrier width (W) is

$$W = (0.566)(X) + 0.61$$

$$W = (0.566)(3.2) + 0.61$$

$$W = 2.4 \text{ m.}$$

3. Use the Varian 90° leakage TVLs for a 20 MV x-ray beam to determine the concrete thickness needed in the secondary wall shown below. Repeat the evaluation for an uncontrolled area.
The barrier transmission factor is given by:

$$B_l = \frac{1000P(d_{sec})^2}{WT}$$

$P = 0.0001$ Sv per week for controlled area

$W = 500$ Gy/wk $\qquad T = 1$ for controlled area

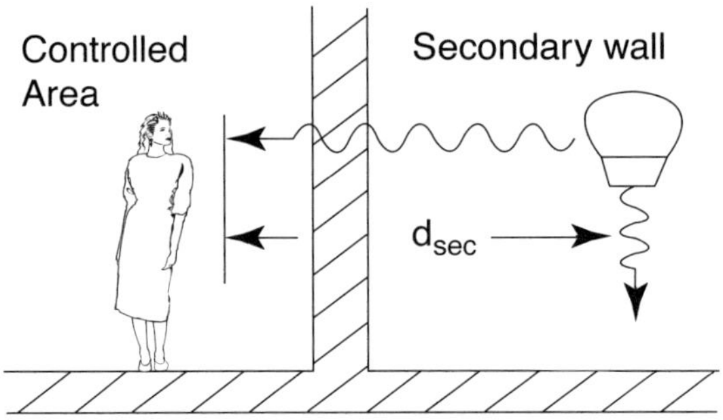

Figure 2-6. Secondary barrier and head leakage radiation

$d_{sec} = 5$ m

P = 0.00002 Sv per week for uncontrolled area

T = 1/4 uncontrolled area.

The barrier transmission factor is:

$$B_1 = \frac{1000(0.0001)(5)^2}{500}$$

$$B_1 = 5 \times 10^{-3} \text{ and } n = \log_{10}(1/B_1) = 2.30.$$

The concrete thickness is S = (n) (TVL)

$$S = (2.30)\ (0.343) = 0.79 \text{ m concrete.}$$

If the area is uncontrolled we have

$$B_1 = \frac{1000(2\times10^{-5})(5)^2}{(500)} = 1.0\times10^{-3}$$

and $n = \log_{10}\ (1.0 \times 10^{-3}) = 3.0$.

The thickness of the wall is

$$S = (3.0)\ (0.343) = 1.03 \text{ m concrete.}$$

Since this is an uncontrolled area, we should now check to see if the dose equivalent outside the wall exceeds 0.02 mSv in any one hour with a workload of 20 Gy in one hour and T equal to one. Solving the barrier transmission equation for P and letting P be the dose equivalent in one hour (D) gives

$$D = \frac{B_l WT}{1000(d^2_{sec})}$$

$$D = \frac{(1.0 \times 10^{-3})(20)(1)}{1000(5^2)} = 0.80 \times 10^{-6} \text{ Sv in one hour}$$

$$= 0.80 \times 10^{-3} \text{ mSv in one hour}$$

So the shielding thickness based on 500 Gy workload in one week will be used.

4. Repeat problem 3 for a 6 MV x-ray beam. Since the beam is less than 10 MV, both patient scatter and head leakage radiation must be considered when designing the secondary barrier. A workload of 1000 Gy per week will be used. The required barrier transmission for patient scatter is given by

$$B_p = \frac{(P)(400/F)(d_{sca})^2(d_{sec})^2}{(a)(W)(T)}$$

where

P = 0.0001 Sv/wk (ALARA controlled area)

F = field area = 40×40 cm^2 (maximum size)

d_{sca} = distance from target to patient = 1 m

d_{sec} = 5 m

a = 0.0006 for 90° scatter

$$B_p = \frac{(0.0001)(400/1600)(1)(5)^2}{(0.0006)(1000)(1)} = 1.04 \times 10^{-3}$$

and $n = 2.98$.

Figure 2-7 (from NCRP Report No. 49) can be used to determine the shielding needed for patient scatter. However, the value of B_p is off the curve. The TVL of the 90° scatter curve is about 0.173 m, so the wall thickness will be

$$S = n \times TVL = 2.98 \times 0.173 = 0.516 \text{ m.}$$

We will now calculate the barrier thickness for head leakage radiation.

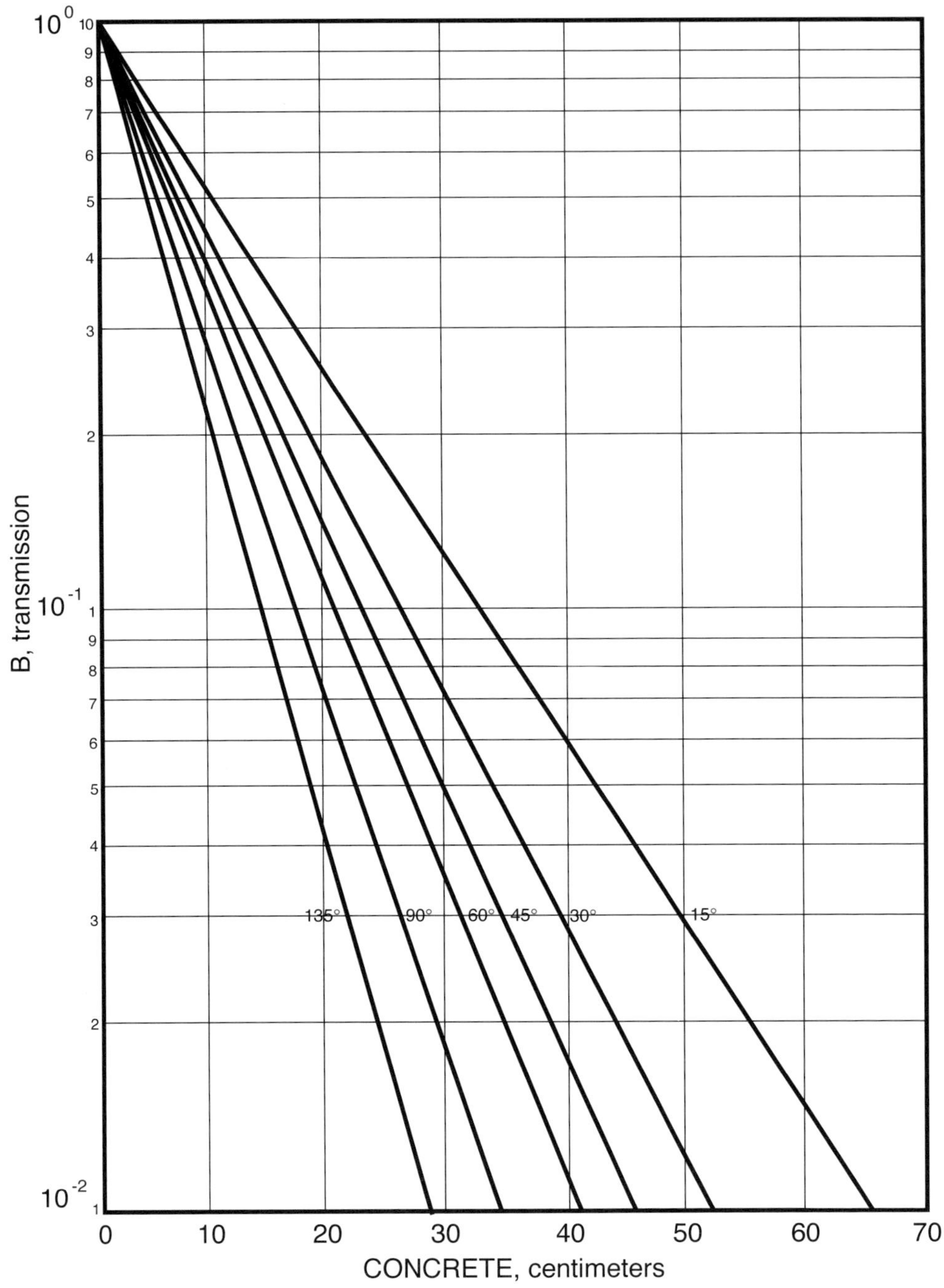

Figure 2-7. Transmission through concrete, density 2.35 g cm^{-3} (147 lb ft^{-3}), for 6 MV primary x-rays scattered at six different angles from a unit density phantom. From NCRP 1976 with permission.

$$B_1 = \frac{(1000)(P)(d^2)}{(W)(T)} = \frac{(1000)(0.0001)(5)^2}{(1000)(1)} = 2.5 \times 10^{-3}$$

and n = 2.60.

The barrier thickness based on head leakage is:

$$S = n \times TVL = 2.60 \times 0.279 = 0.725 \text{ m concrete.}$$

We could use 0.725/6.2 = 0.12 m lead in place of concrete or 0.725/3.5 = 0.21 m steel. The difference between the thickness for head leakage and patient scatter is 0.209 m, which is less than three HVL. To be on the safe side, one HVL of concrete will be added to the larger S to give 0.81 m concrete.

5. Design a tapered lead primary barrier for placement on top of a one-foot-thick concrete slab as shown in figure 2-8. Ignore any problems created by neutrons produced in the lead slab. The accelerator operates at 18 MeV, and the maximum beam size at the isocenter is 40 × 40 cm^2. The area above the machine is to be uncontrolled with an occupancy factor of 1/16, and the use factor is 1/4 for the vertical up direction. The use factor for other gantry angles when the beam intercepts the ceiling barrier is 1/10. The room dimensions are given in feet, which is a common unit for room plans in the United States.

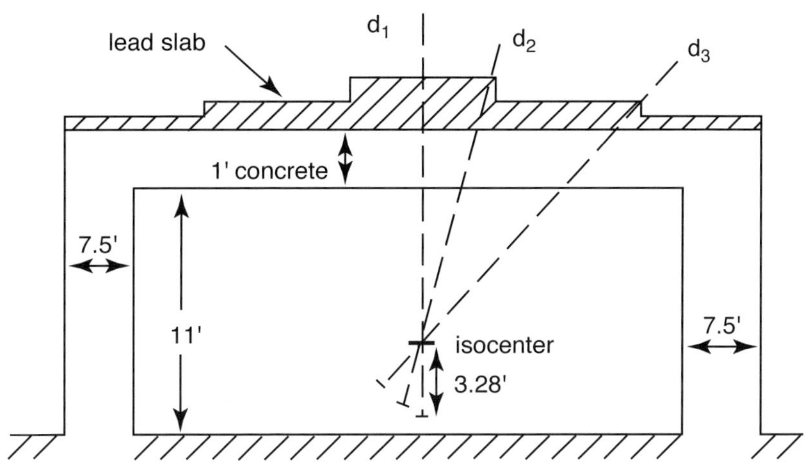

Figure 2-8. Tapered metal ceiling barrier. The isocenter is 1.3 m off the floor.

The barrier transmission factor is calculated starting with the center section.

$$B_X = \frac{Pd_1^2}{WUT} = \frac{(2\times 10^{-5})(3.65)^2}{(500)(1/4)(1/16)} = 3.41 \times 10^{-5}$$

and n = 4.47

Note that d_1 is the distance from the target to 0.305 m above the shield in meters, and the distance from the floor to the isocenter is 1.3 m. However, in order to simplify the problem the thickness of the lead has been ignored in determining d_1. If the shield were all concrete, the thickness would be

$$S = n \times TVL = 4.47 \times 0.444 \text{ m} = 1.98 \text{ m concrete.}$$

We already have 0.305 m of concrete, so lead equivalent to 1.67 m of concrete is required. The approximate thickness of lead (S_1') is given below. The value 0.056 is the TVL for lead at 18 MV.

$$S_1' = (1.67/0.444)(0.056) = 0.211 \text{ m lead}$$

Equations 2-1 and 2-5 will now be used to obtain a more accurate evaluation of the lead thickness S_1.

$$B_X = \frac{Pd_1^2}{WUT} \qquad\qquad n = \text{Log}\ (1/B_x)$$

Substituting equation 2-1 into equation 2-5 gives the following:

$$n = \log\ (WUT/Pd_1^2)$$

n is also given by: $n = S_1/0.056 + 0.305/0.444$.

Equating the two equations for n gives:

$$S_1/0.056 + 0.305/0.444 = \log(WUT/Pd_1^2)$$

The new value of d_1 is 3.65 m plus S_1'.

$$S_1/0.56 + 0.035/0.444 = \log\ [WUT/P(3.65 + S_1')^2]$$

Since the log term varies slowly with S_1', one can obtain the lead thickness (S_1) to three significant figures from the above equation. Based on the value of 0.211 m for S_1', a value of 0.209 m is found for S_1. The lead thickness will be rounded off to 0.21 m, and the new value of the distance from the target to 0.305 m above the shield (d_1) is 3.86 m.

Next the length (L_1) and width (W_1) of the center lead section of the shield are calculated based on figure 2-9.

$$L_1 = W_1 = (0.566)\ (X_2) + 0.61 \text{ m}$$

The distance X_2 cannot be determined with the present information. However, X_2 is approximately equal to X_1.

$$L_1 = W_1 \cong (0.566)\ (X_1) + 0.61 \text{ m}$$

where $X_1 = d_1 - S_1 - 0.305 = 3.86 - 0.21 - 0.305 = 3.35$ m

and $L_1 = W_1 \cong 2.51$ m

The value of X_2 in meters can now be approximated by the following. Distance C is the distance from the isocenter to the metal slab (see figure 2-9).

$$X_2 = \sqrt{(L_1/2)^2 + C_1^2} + 1.0 = \sqrt{(2.51/2)^2 + 2.35^2} + 1.0 \text{ m}$$

$$X_2 = 3.66 \text{ m}$$

The length and width of the lead section are evaluated a second time using X_2.

$$L_1 = W_1 = (0.566)\ (3.66) + 0.61 = 2.68 \text{ M}$$

The length (L) of the remaining sections of lead are each made 1.83 m (6').

The lead thickness of the second section is based on an approximation of the distance d_2.

$$d_2 \cong X_2 + S_1 + 0.305 = 4.17 \text{ m}$$

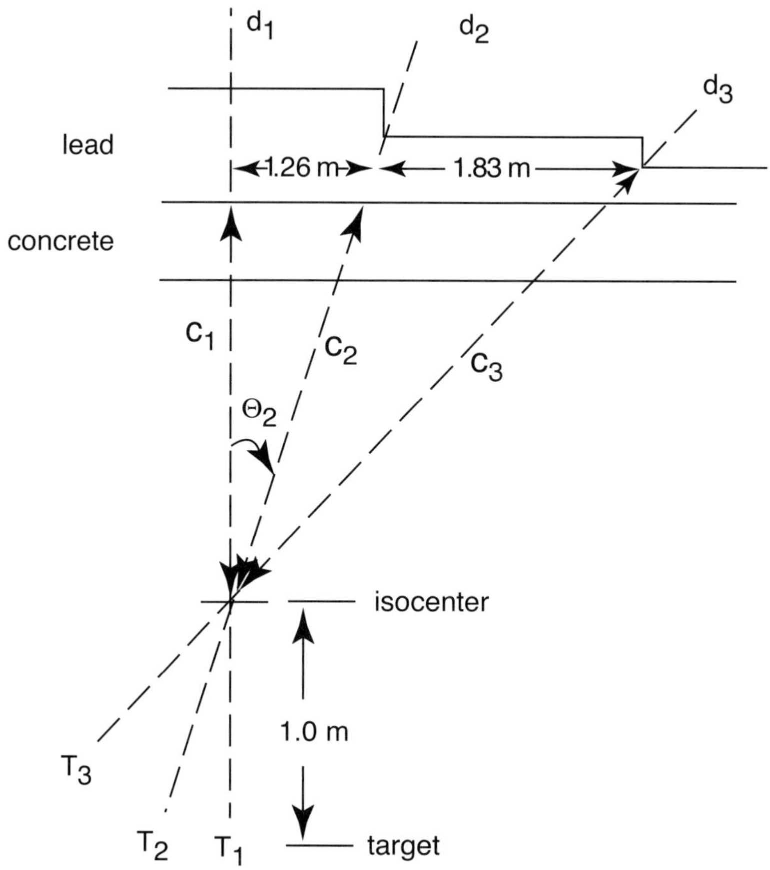

Figure 2-9. Section view of tapered ceiling shield

The barrier transmission factor for the second lead segment is

$$B = \frac{Pd_2^2}{WUT} = \frac{(2 \times 10^{-5})(4.17)^2}{(500)(1/10)(1/16)} = 1.11 \times 10^{-4}$$

and $\quad n = 3.95$

$$\theta_2 = \text{Tan}^{-1}\ [(L_1/2)/C_1\ ] = \text{Tan}^{-1}(1.26/2.35) = 28.2^\circ$$

The slant thickness of concrete (S) is evaluated using θ_2.

$$S\ = 0.305/\cos\ (28.2^\circ) = 0.346 \text{ m concrete}$$

This thickness of concrete is equivalent to 0.78 TVL, and the number of lead TVL needed is given by

$$n = 3.95 - 0.78 = 3.17.$$

The required thickness of lead is

$$S_2 = (3.17)\ (0.056) = 0.18 \text{ m}.$$

The width of the second lead segment is based on the value of X_3.

$$X_3 = \sqrt{C_1^2 + (L_1/2 + L_2)^2} + 1.0 \text{ m}$$

$$X_3 = \sqrt{(2.35)^2 + (2.68/2 + 1.83)^2} + 1 \text{ m}$$

$$X_3 = 4.95\text{m}$$

and

$$W_2 = (0.566)\ (4.95) + 0.61 = 3.41 \text{ m}$$

The same procedure would be used for the remaining sections of the lead portion of the barrier. Note that chapter 6 covers the problems created by neutrons produced when the beam strikes the lead barrier.

Problems

1. The primary wall for the 20 MeV accelerator in example 1 of this chapter must be changed to 3' concrete plus another material. Distance d is to remain unchanged.
   a. How much lead will be needed?
   b. If steel is used in place of lead, what thickness is required?
   c. How much earth would be needed? (Use a value of 18 MV.)

2. Calculate the dose rate outside the wall barrier if the accelerator is operated at 400 cGy/min at the isocenter.

3. Evaluate the dose outside the barrier in any one hour of operation based on a workload of 2000 cGy in one hour of operation.

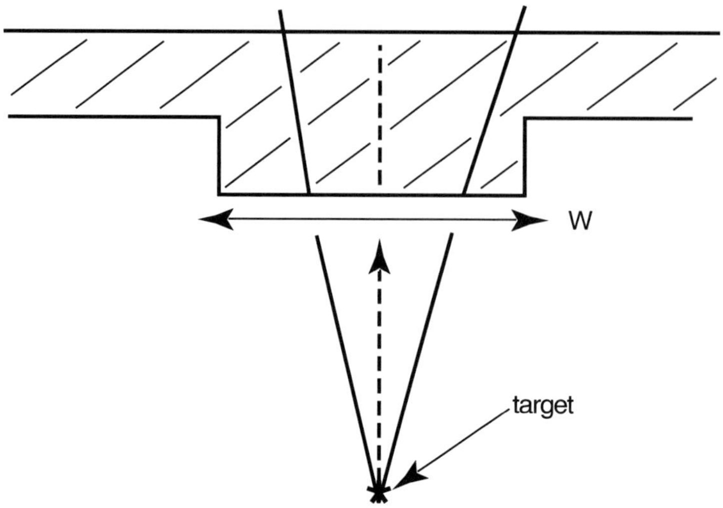

Figure 2-10. Ceiling primary barrier

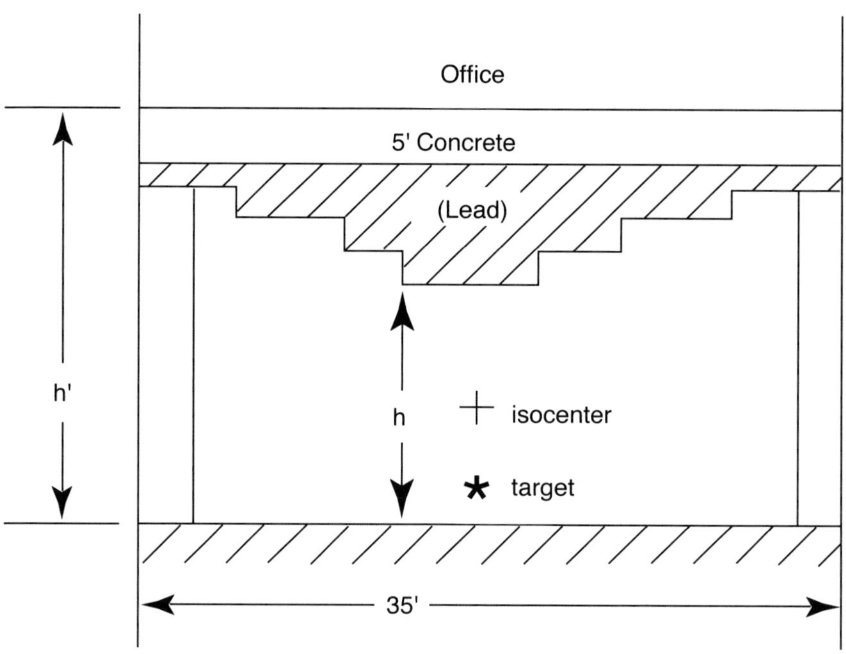

Figure 2-11. Tapered lead and concrete ceiling barrier

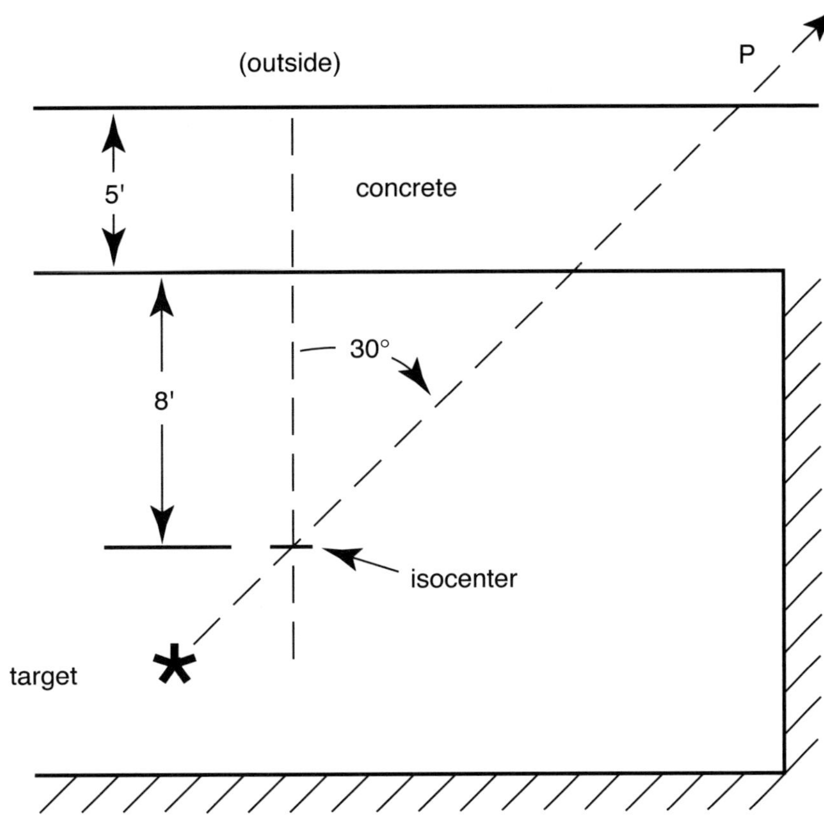

Figure 2-12. Angled beam

4. Evaluate the width (W) of the primary wall barrier (see figure 2-10) if the shield protrudes into the treatment room for the 20 MeV accelerator in example 1 of this chapter. The room height from the floor to the ceiling slab is 11', and the isocenter is 4.26' off the floor. Assume the primary ceiling slab is 6.5' thick. State all assumptions made.

5. A ceiling slab is to contain lead and concrete (5') for an 18 MeV accelerator (see figure 2-11). The workload is 1×10^5 cGy per week and h′ = 17.5'. Make length L_2 equal to 6'. Carry out the following calculations and list all assumptions used.
   a. Calculate lead thicknesses.
   b. Evaluate length of lead slab in the plane of target rotation.
   c. Evaluate the width of each lead slab.

6. The gantry of an 18 MeV accelerator is angled 30° off vertical as shown in figure 2-12. Evaluate the dose rate to be expected outside the shield at Point P. What is the dose at point P per week of operation if the workload is 1×10^5 cGy/week, the use factor for the 30° angle is 1/20, and T = 1/16? Assume that the workload in any one hour of operation is 2000 cGy. Calculate the dose in one hour of operation at Point P. Assume U = T = 1 for the calculation.

7. Calculate the barrier thickness and dose levels for the following locations in the 18 MeV accelerator room shown in figures 2-13 and 2-14. Note that all barriers are ordinary concrete and the scale of the room drawing is shown by the one m marker. Only the outer room dimensions are to scale.
   a. Wall thickness for primary north wall
   b. Ceiling thickness (primary)
   c. West wall (secondary)
   d. Ceiling thickness (secondary)
   e. East wall (secondary)

   Operating conditions:
   Workload in any one hour = 2000 cGy
   U = T = 1 (for one hour evaluation)
   Workload = 1×10^5 cGy of 18 MV x-ray per week
   Walls and ceiling are ordinary concrete (147 lb/ft^3)
   Floor is a concrete slab on grade

Primary Barriers

Location	*Adjoining area*	*T*	*Type of area**	*U*
North wall	outside	1/8	U	1/4
South wall	stretcher waiting	1	C	1/4
Ceiling	outside	1/16	U	1/4

*U = uncontrolled area, C = controlled area

Secondary Barriers

Location	*Adjoining area*	*T*	*Type of area**
West wall	console	1	C
East wall	work room	1	C
North wall	outside	1/8	U
South wall	stretcher waiting	1	C
Ceiling	outside	1/16	U

*U = uncontrolled area, C = controlled area

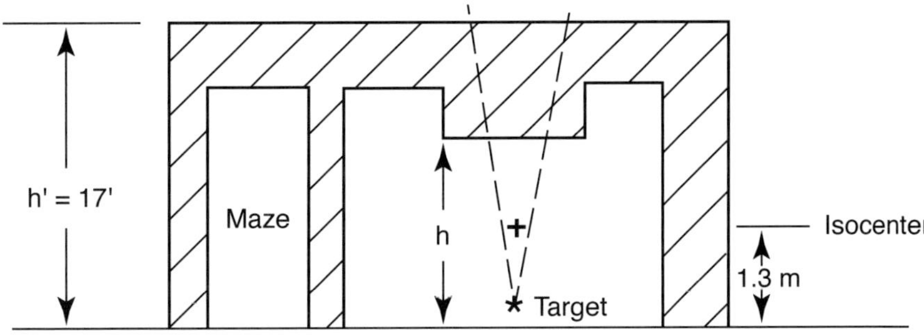

Figure 2-13. Section view of treatment room. View in plane perpendicular to the target rotational plane. Not to scale.

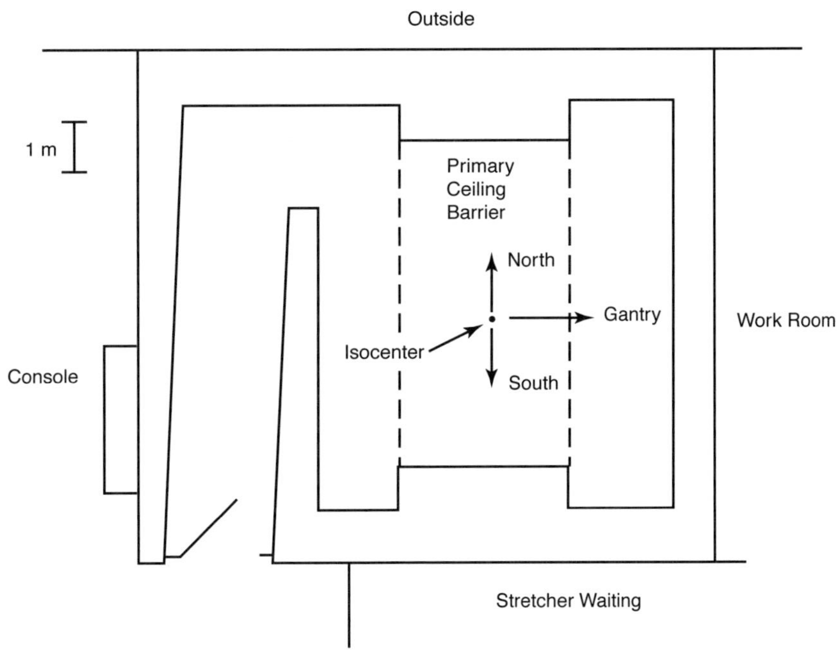

Figure 2-14. Floor plan of treatment room. Note 1 m scale mark.

8. Calculate the thickness of concrete needed for the north wall secondary barrier of figure 2-14 for a 25 MeV accelerator. Use the TVL values given in Table 2-7 for head leakage at an angle of 35° and take into consideration the slant thickness.

3

Conventional Maze Design

A maze such as the one shown in figure 3-1 is typically used to reduce the radiation level at the entrance of the accelerator room so that a massive door is not required. In this chapter mazes for low-energy treatment rooms ($\leq$ 10 MeV) will be discussed. A typical treatment room door consists of a sheet of lead 0.6 to 1.0 cm thick placed at the center of a 5 cm thick solid core wood door. If floor space is at a premium, the maze can be eliminated and a direct shielded door equivalent to a secondary barrier substituted (McGinley 1993).

The radiation reaching the maze door is due to scattering from the room surfaces and patient, as well as direct penetration of radiation through the maze wall (D′ of figure 3-1). The scattered radiation reaching the maze door is made up of the following components:

1. Primary beam scattered from room surfaces (S_s)
2. Head leakage photons scattered by room surfaces (L)
3. Primary scatter from the patient (S_p)

The radiation scattered to the door when the primary beam strikes wall C of figure 3-1 can be calculated by use of equation 3-1, which is presented in NCRP Report No. 51 (NCRP 1977).

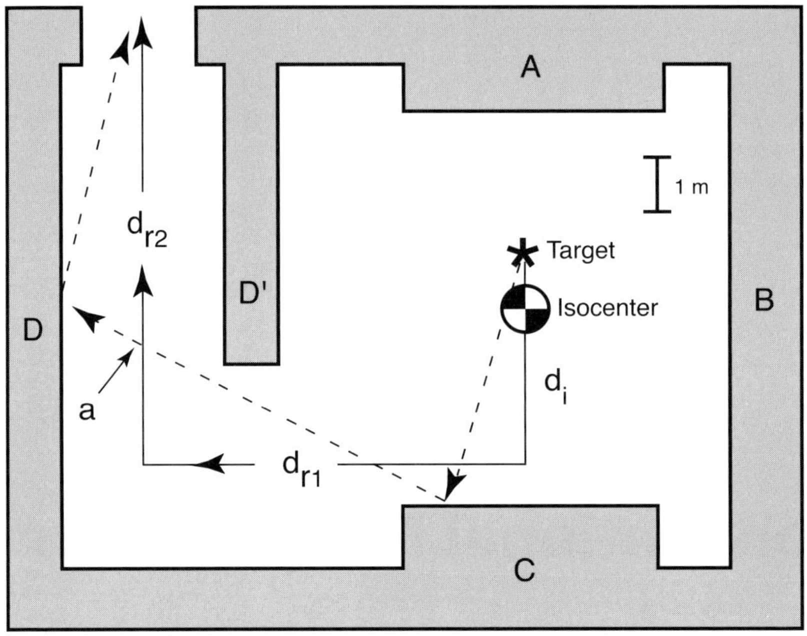

Figure 3-1. Treatment room floor plan for maze calculation

$$S_s = \frac{D_0\ \alpha_1\ A_1\ \alpha_2\ A_2}{(d_i d_{r1} d_{r2})^2} \tag{3-1}$$

where

S_s = dose at door

D_0 = workload of accelerator

α_1 = reflection coefficient at first reflection based on a beam energy of one-half the megavoltage of the accelerator

A_1 = beam area at first reflection (m^2)

α_2 = reflection coefficient at second reflection based on an energy of 0.5 MeV

A_2 = cross section of maze (m^2)

d_i = distance from the target to the first reflection (m)

d_{r1} = centerline distance along first leg of maze (m)

d_{r2} = centerline distance along second leg of maze (m).

Morgan et al. (1995) have found that equation 3-1 gives results that are too small by a factor of as much as ten for a 6 MeV accelerator. The largest difference between the measured and calculated values was obtained when the beam irradiated the wall adjacent to the maze opening, as shown in figure 3-1. It was also reported (Morgan et al. 1995) that the peak energy of the x-ray spectrum at the outer maze entrance is approximately 0.2 MeV. Therefore, a portion of the underestimation of the dose by equation 3-1 may be due to the lower value of α_2 obtained by assuming the average energy of the scattered radiation is 0.5 MeV. McGinley and James (1997) have investigated the accuracy of equation 3-1 for a 6 and a 10 MeV medical accelerator room and agree with Morgan et al. that the method described in NCRP Report No. 51 to evaluate the radiation scattered from the treatment room wall predicts a radiation dose that is less than the measured value. It was also confirmed by McGinley and James (1997) that the average energy of the radiation field at the outer maze entrance was on the order of 0.2 MeV.

Numark and Kase (1985) have modified the technique given in NCRP Report No. 51 for wall scatter and report agreement between calculations derived from the modified method and actual measurements within a factor of two. The average energy of the primary beam was assigned a value of one-third the megavoltage as opposed to one-half the megavoltage as suggested in NCRP Report No. 51. The angle of the reflected radiation was determined by a line extending from the beam center at the wall to point a of figure 3-2. As can be seen from figure 3-2, α_1, α_2, d_{r1}, and d_{r2} will take on values differing from those assigned when the NCRP technique is used. McGinley and James (1997) employed the method used by Numark and Kase for facilities housing 6 and 10 MeV accelerators and found agreement within a factor of two with measured values. The following restrictions apply for equation 3-1. The height to width ratio of the maze must be between one and two, and the value of $d_{r2}/(A_2)^{1/2}$ must be between two and six. It has been the author's experience that the second requirement is not met by a high percentage of low-energy accelerator rooms due to the relatively short length of the maze.

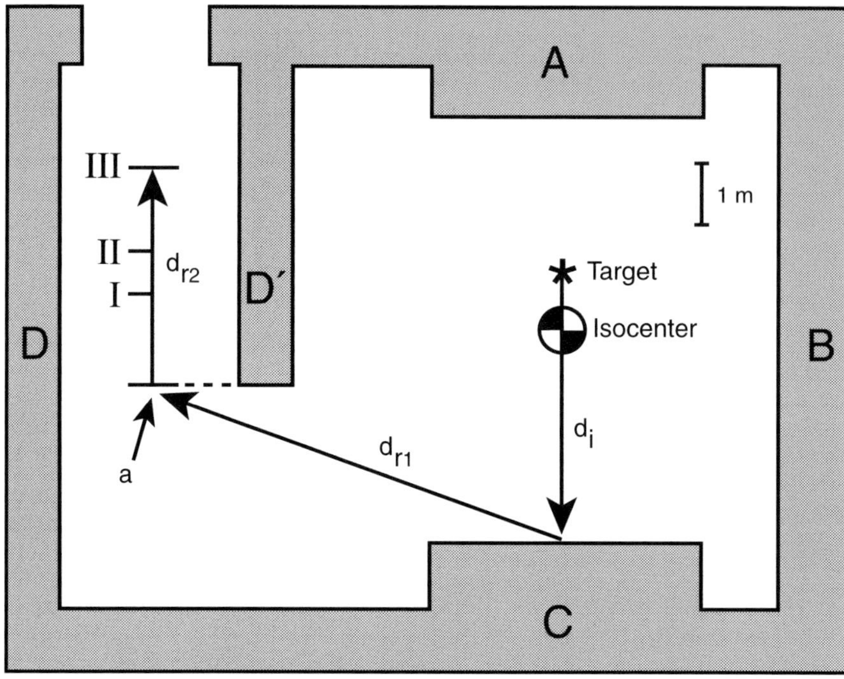

Figure 3-2. Room diagram for wall scatter (S_s). Based on Numark and Kase (1985).

Values of the reflection coefficient may be obtained from figure 3-3, which was reproduced from NCRP Report No. 51 for photons with energy between 0.1 and 10 MeV in concrete, lead, and iron. Only two scattering geometries are presented in NCRP Report No. 51 that can be used to select the reflection coefficient—one for normal incidence of the beam on the scattering surface and one for equal angle of incidence and reflection. For a typical room one or both scattering conditions may not apply, leading to uncertainty in the reflection coefficient. For photon energies above 10 MeV, the 10 MeV reflection coefficient is used. This procedure is considered to be a conservative estimation of the radiation level at the outer door.

Head leakage radiation that strikes wall C as shown in figure 3-4 can undergo a single scatter and reach the maze door. This radiation is more penetrating than the doubly scattered primary beam and the patient scatter and has an average energy of approximately 0.3 MeV at the maze door for a 6 MeV accelerator. Equation 3-1 is modified as shown below for the calculation of the head leakage reaching the door after a single scatter.

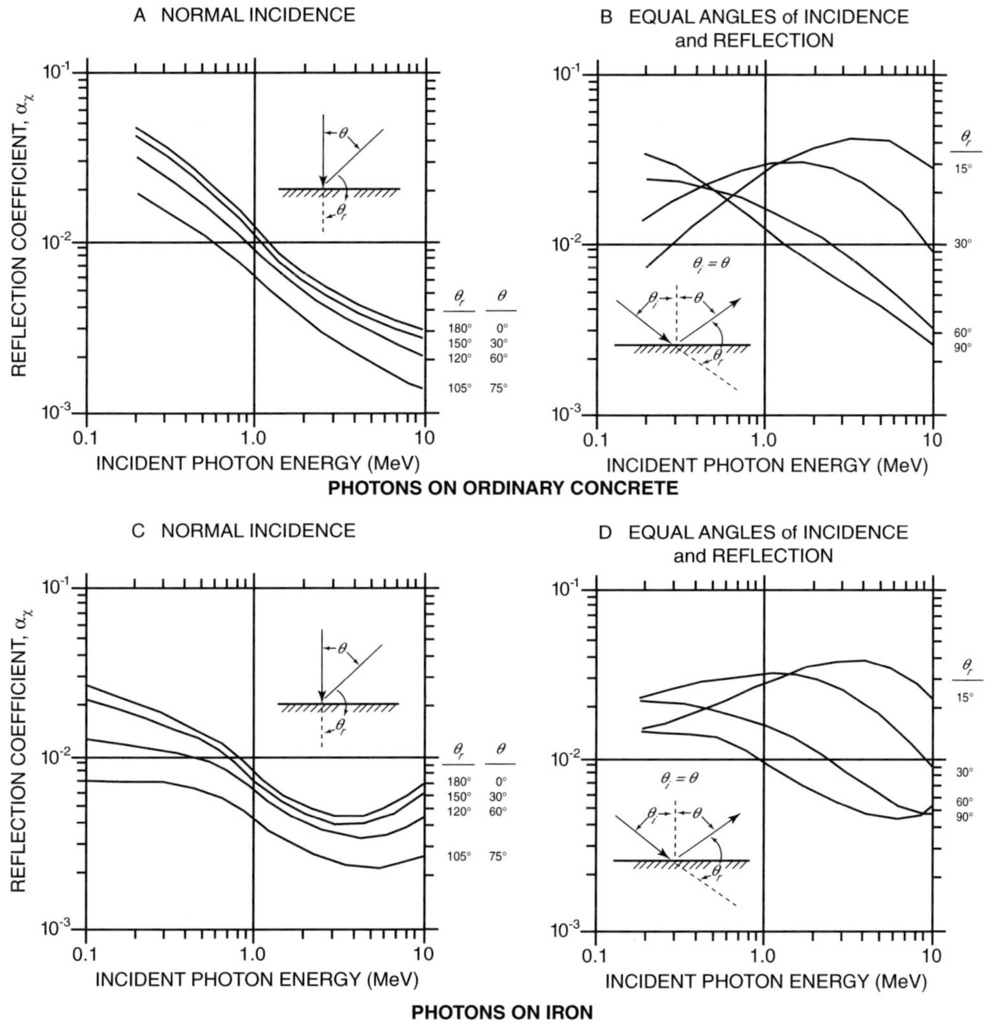

Figure 3-3. Reflection coefficients for various materials. Reprinted with permission from NCRP Report No. 51 (NCRP 1977).

$$L = \frac{L_0 \, D_0 \, \alpha_1 \, A_1}{(d_s d_i)^2} \tag{3-2}$$

where

L = dose at the maze door due to head leakage

L_0 = ratio of dose due to head leakage at 1.0 m from the target to the dose at the isocenter

D_0 = workload of accelerator

α_1 = reflection coefficient for wall reflection

A_1 = area of wall C that can be seen from the maze door (m^2)

d_i = distance from the target to the maze centerline (m)

d_s = centerline distance along the maze (m).

Agreement within a factor of two of measured and calculated dose values was found by McGinley and James (1997) when equation 3-2 was used to establish the head leakage radiation scattered to the maze outer entrance for 6 and 10 MeV accelerators. For these calculations, the head leakage was based on measured values as opposed to the accepted value of 0.001 or 0.1%. In some cases, the measured head leakage may be a factor of four times smaller than the accepted values. The beam directions used by McGinley and James (1997) were vertical down, vertical up, beam horizontal on wall C, and beam horizontal on wall A of figure 3-4. The energy assigned to the head leakage radiation as it emerged from the accelerator was obtained from the results reported by Nelson and LaRiviere (1984) for 6 and 10 MeV medical accelerators. Values of 1.4 and 1.5 MeV were used for the

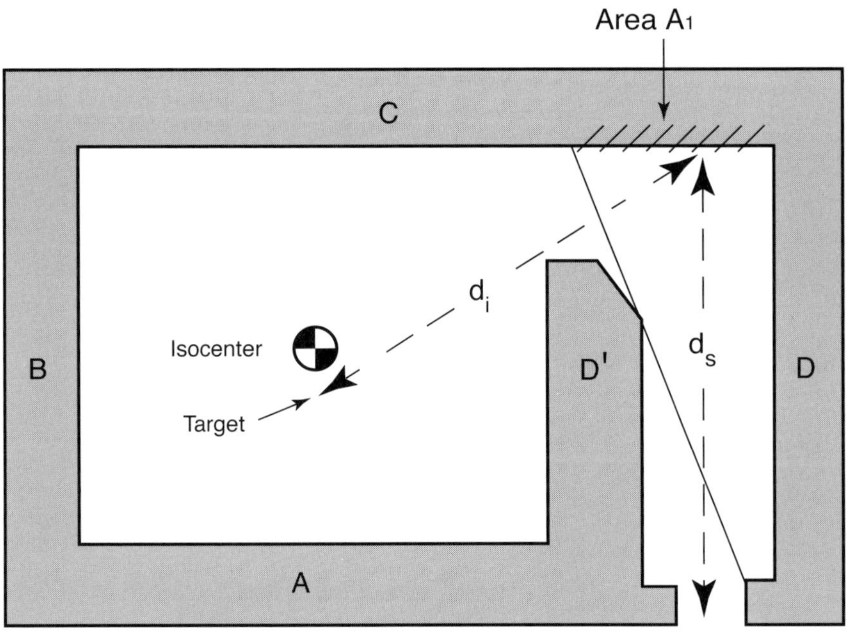

Figure 3-4. Path of head leakage scatter to maze door

average energy of the head leakage radiation produced by the 6 and 10 MeV accelerator, respectively. These energies correspond to the values expected for leakage radiation leaving the accelerator along line d_i of figure 3-4. The reflection coefficient α_1 is based on the value of the radiation energy mentioned above.

Patient scatter to the maze door is calculated by use of equation 3-3 for accelerators with an energy ≤10 MeV. When the energy of the accelerator is greater than 10 MeV, patient scatter can be ignored. Figure 3-5 depicts the parameters used in equation 3-3 to calculate the radiation scattered by the patient to the maze door.

$$S_p = \frac{aD_0\ (F/400)\alpha_1 A_1}{(d_{sca} d_{sec}\, d_{r1})^2} \tag{3-3}$$

where

S_p = dose at maze door due to patient scatter

a = reflection coefficient for patient from Table 2-1

D_0 = workload of accelerator

F = field area at patient (cm^2)

α_1 = reflection coefficient for wall reflection (E = 0.5 MeV)

A_1 = area (m^2) of maze back wall that can be seen from outer maze entrance

d_{sca} = distance from target to patient (m)

d_{sec} = distance from patient to maze centerline (m)

d_{rl} = centerline distance along maze (m).

The radiation transmitted through maze wall D′ of figure 3-1 to the treatment room door is evaluated by use of equation 3-4 and compared with the radiation scattered down the maze to the door.

$$T = \frac{L_0\, D_0\, B}{(d'')^2} \tag{3-4}$$

where

B = barrier transmission factor for wall D′

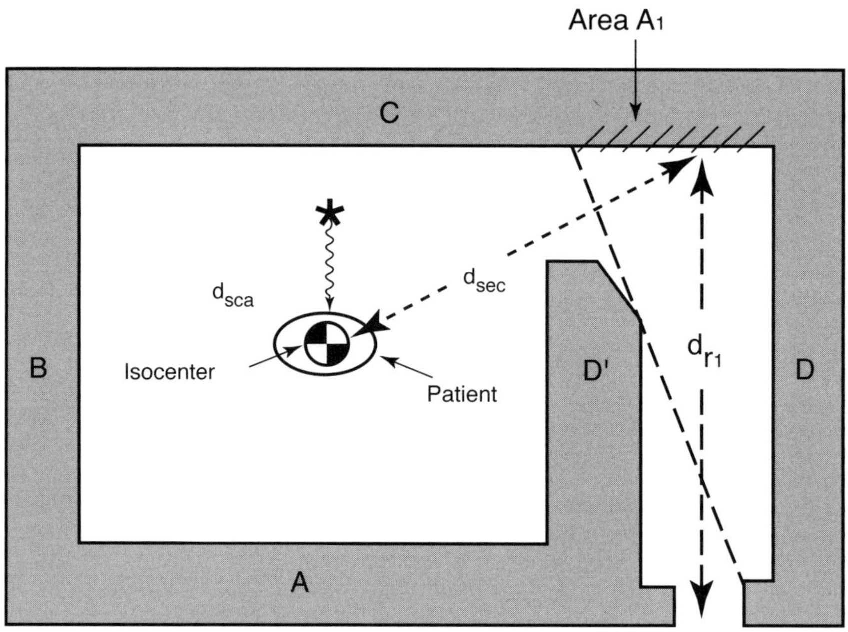

Figure 3-5. Path of patient scatter to maze door

d″ = distance from the target to the center of the maze door.

The maximum dose at the maze door is produced by aiming the beam toward wall C of figure 3-1 with the collimator fully open and a patient in the beam (McGinley and James 1997). The dose (D_c) from all components (S_S, S_p, L, and T) of the radiation field at the maze door when the beam irradiates wall C is given by equation 3-5. Note that the workload with the beam aimed at wall C is used to calculate the dose components.

$$D_c = S_p + f(S_s) + L + T \qquad (3\text{-}5)$$

where

f = fraction of beam transmitted through patient

Values of the patient transmission factor (f) of 0.23 for a 6 MV x-ray beam and 0.27 for a 10 MV beam have been reported by McGinley and James (1997). Note that in equation 3-5 it has been assumed that the portion of the primary beam scattered from the room surfaces has been reduced by a factor (f) equivalent to the beam transmitted through the patient.

For the typical case in which the use factors (U) for the major beam directions (up, down, horizontal on wall A and C) are each 1/4 the total dose (D_t) at the maze door, the following equation is given. This equation is to be used for rooms with a floor plan similar to that shown in figure 3-1.

$$D_t = 2.64\ D_c \tag{3-6}$$

The transmission factor required for the door shielding is calculated by dividing D_t into the protection level needed for the area outside the door. Once the transmission has been evaluated, the thickness of lead needed in the door for a 6 MeV accelerator can be determined from the curves shown in figure 3-6. These curves are arranged according to the maze length distance, d_{r2}, of figure 3-2. For a 10 MeV accelerator, equation 3-6 still applies and the lead thickness for the door can be based on broad beam data for 0.21 MeV photons (McGinley and James 1997).

When the energy of the accelerator is above 10 MeV, the techniques outlined above for evaluating the radiation field at the outer maze entrance are still valid. However, the presence of photoneutrons and capture gamma rays must be considered as discussed in chapters 4 and 5.

Example Calculations

1. Evaluate the maximum dose per week at the maze door for the 6 MeV accelerator room described below. The walls are constructed of concrete, and the workload is 1×10^5 cGy per week at the isocenter. The room and maze heights are 3.35 m, and the beam size is $0.40 \times 0.40\ m^2$ at the isocenter. The beam transmission through the patient is 0.23. The use factor for the beam aimed at wall C is one-fourth. Therefore, the workload with the beam on wall C is 2.5×10^4 cGy per week. From the room diagram, the following dimensions are determined.

   maze width = 2.4 m
   maze wall slant thickness = 0.91 m
   d_{r1} = 5.8 m (wall scatter)
   d_{r1} = 4.9 m (patient scatter)
   d_{r2} = 2.4 m

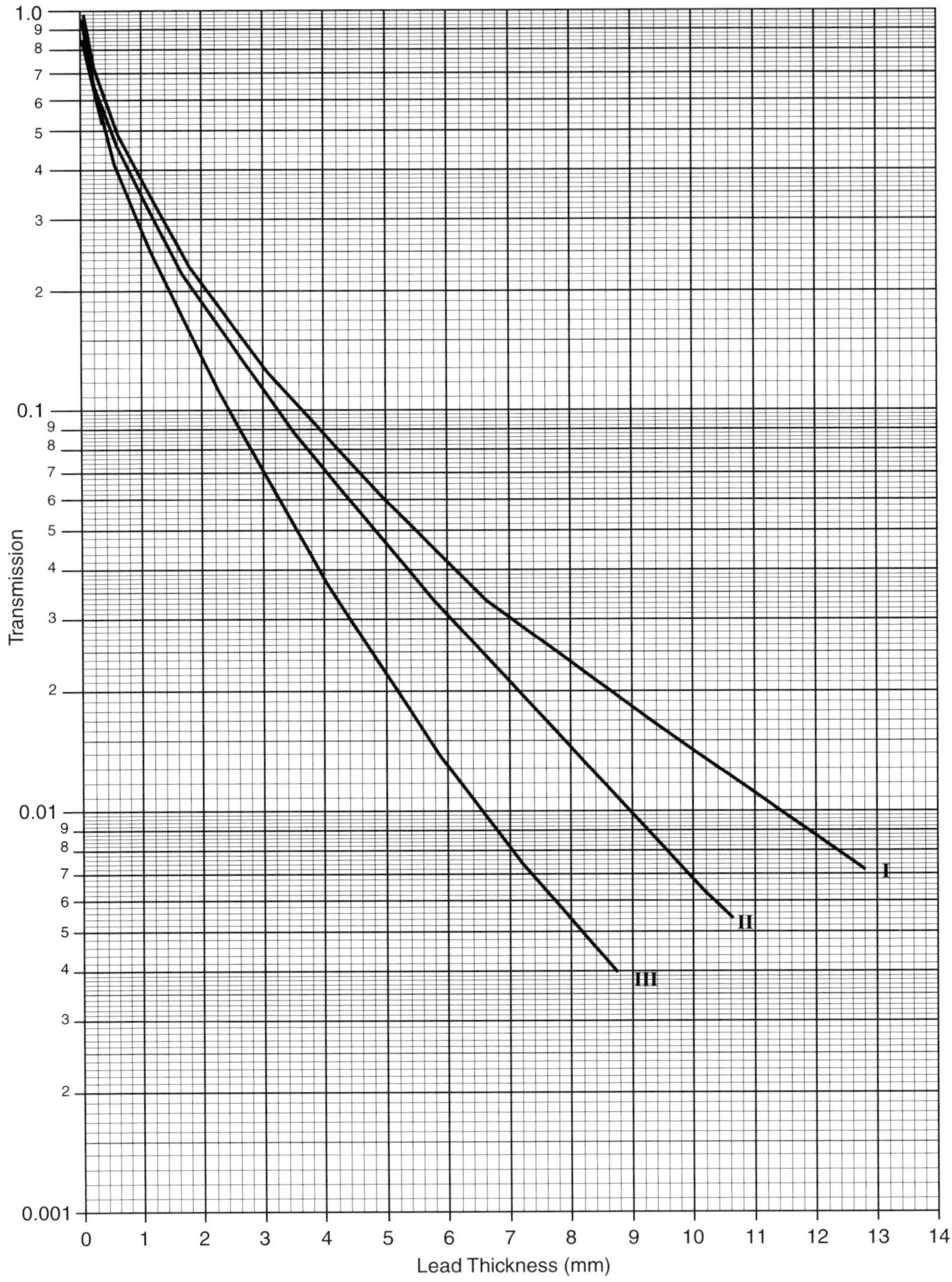

Figure 3-6. Transmission through lead of the radiation field in the maze of a 6 MeV accelerator facility with the beam aimed at wall C. The maze lengths for curves I, II, and III are 1.5 m, 2.0 m, and 3.4 m, respectively.

$d_i = 4.0$ m
$d_s = 5.9$ m
$d_1 = 3.5$ m
$A_1 = 2.56\ m^2$ (wall scatter)
$d_{sca} = 1$ m
$d_{sec} = 6.1$ m
$A_1 = 14.3\ m^2$ (patient and head leakage scatter)

a. Patient scatter

From equation 3-3 we have

$$S_p = \frac{aD_0\,(F/400)\alpha_1 A_1}{(d_{sca}\,d_{sec}\,d_{r1})^2}$$

$$S_p = \frac{(0.00075)(2.5\times 10^4)(1600/400)(0.02)(14.3)}{(1\times 6.1\times 4.9)^2}$$

$S_p = 0.0237$ cGy per week = 23.7 mrem per week.

b. Wall scatter

The wall scatter is based on the 23% transmission of the primary beam through the patient.

From equation 3-1 we have:

$$S_s = \frac{D_0\,\alpha_1\,A_1\,\alpha_2\,A_2}{(d_i d_{r1} d_{r2})^2}$$

$$S_s = \frac{(2.5\times 10^4)(0.005)(2.56)(0.02)(8.0)}{(4.0\times 5.8\times 2.4)^2}$$

$S_s = 0.0165$ cGy per week = 16.5 mrem per week.

Correcting for the patient transmission (f) gives

S_s = (16.5 mrem per week) (0.23) = 3.8 mrem per week.

c. Head Leakage

Direct measurements give a value of 0.03% head leakage on a line from the target to the inner maze entrance. We will use an energy of 1.4 MeV for the leakage. Equation 3-2 gives:

$$L = \frac{L_0 D_0 \alpha_1 A_1}{(d_s d_1)^2}$$

$$L = 0.0025 \text{ cGy per week} = 2.5 \text{ mrem per week.}$$

d. Maze wall transmission

We will assume that the head leakage is attenuated in the maze wall with a TVL of 0.279 m concrete.

$$T = (\text{leakage})\ (D_0)\ (10^{-\#TVL})\ (1/d)^2$$

The number of TVLs is 0.91/0.279 = 3.26 and the distance from the target to the maze door is 5.5 m.

$$T = (0.0003)\ (2.5 \times 10^4)\ (10^{-3.26})\ (1/5.5)^2$$

$$T = 0.000125 \text{ cGy per week} = 0.125 \text{ mrem per week}$$

e. The dose per week with the beam on wall C is:

$$D_c = \text{patient scatter} + \text{wall scatter} + \text{head leakage scatter} + \text{maze wall transmission}$$

$$D_c = 23.7 + 3.8 + 2.5 + 0.12 = 30 \text{ mrem per week.}$$

f. The total dose per week for the major beam angles is given by equation 3-6.

$$D_t = 2.64\ D_c$$

$$D_t = (2.64)\ (30) = 79.2 \text{ mrem per week}$$

2. Determine how much lead shielding is needed in the door to reduce the dose per week to the ALARA level (10 mrem per week). The required transmission is:

$$B = 10/79.2 = 0.126.$$

From figure 3-6 we find that 3 mm of lead is required for the door. This is a conservative evaluation of the door shielding requirements because the scattered radiation will be reduced in intensity for other beam directions.

Problem

Repeat example 1 and 2 based on the following room diagram. The room and maze ceiling heights are 3.35 m each.

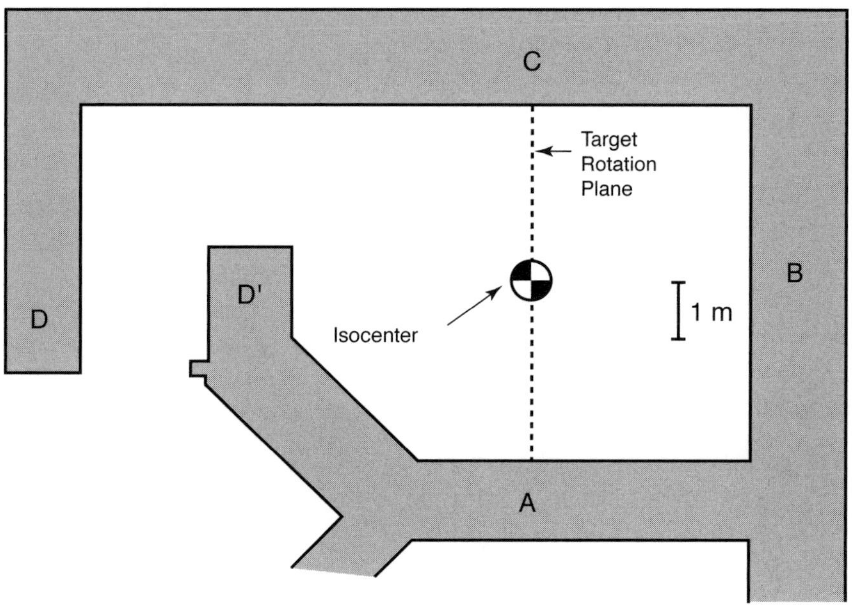

Figure 3-7. Floor plan of a treatment room with a 6 MeV accelerator

4

Photoneutrons

Photoneutron Production

Medical electron accelerators operating above 10 MeV produce radiation beams that are contaminated with neutrons. Therefore, shielding plans for high-energy accelerator rooms must consider the neutron component of the radiation field. Figure 4-1 is a simplified diagram showing the major parts of the accelerator from which neutrons are generated. Photon interactions result in neutrons being ejected from the nucleus of atoms making up the parts of the accelerator shown in figure 4-1.

These neutrons are referred to as photoneutrons, and the reaction is diagrammed below. A similar reaction can occur with electrons, but the

$$^{A}X(\gamma,n)^{A-1}X$$

neutron yield is several orders of magnitude lower than that for the photon reaction and, therefore, will be ignored. Neutrons are also produced by the $(\gamma,2n)$ and the (γ,pn) reaction, but the yield is low compared with the (γ,n) reaction.

Extensive measurements of the cross sections of photoneutron interactions have been reported as a function of the photon energy

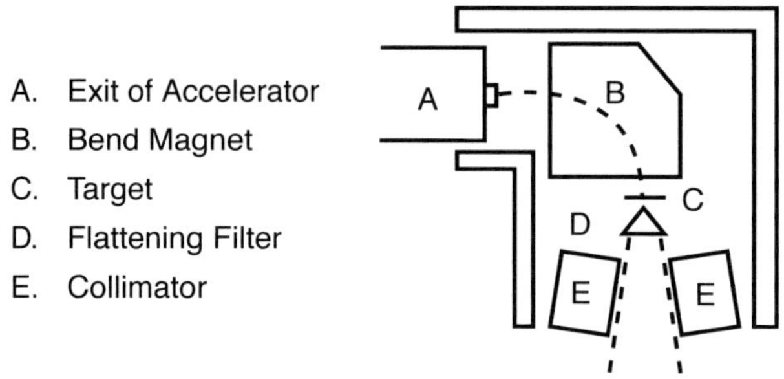

Figure 4-1. Simplified diagram of the electron accelerator

(Berman 1976). Figure 4-2 shows the general shape of the cross-section curve for medium and high atomic number materials. The cross-section curve has a threshold energy (E_t) below which the (γ,n) reaction does not occur. Table 4-1 lists the minimum threshold energy based on the isotopes that make up various metals found in medical accelerators. The cross-section curve has a peak 3-7 MeV above the threshold energy and then falls off with increasing energy. The peak located at photon energy E_m is called a giant resonance peak.

Table 4-1 Minimum threshold energy for the (g,n) reaction in metals*

Element	*Atomic weight*	*Abundance (%)*	*Threshold Energy (MeV)*
A1	27	100	13.1
Fe	54	5.8	13.4
Cu	65	30.8	9.91
W	183	14.3	6.19
Pb	207	22.1	6.74

*Adapted from NCRP 1984.

The yield of photoneutrons depends on the material and the photon energy. Table 4-2 contains relative neutron yields calculated from data given in NCRP Report Number 79 (NCRP 1984). The values in Table 4-2 have been normalized to one for tungsten at 25 MeV. The target material is assumed to be bombarded by electrons, which generate an electromagnetic shower, and the photons undergo (γ,n) reactions in the material. The target is semi-infinite thick, which means that it is thick enough to stop the electromagnetic shower but thin

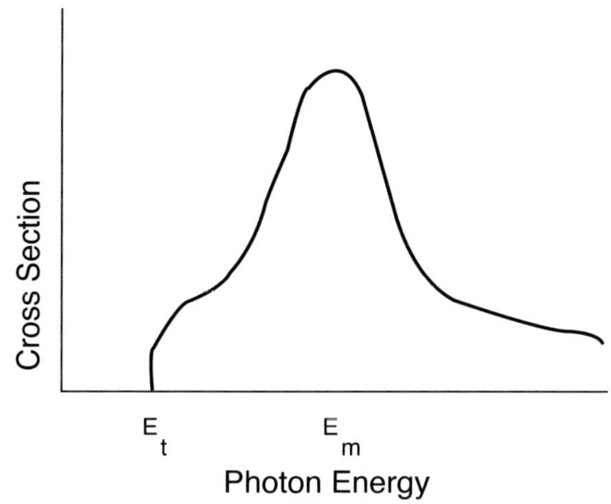

Figure 4-2. Photoneutron cross-section curve

enough that no neutrons are absorbed in the target. As can be seen in Table 4-2, the most common materials (lead and tungsten) in the accelerator head have high photoneutron yields. The photoneutrons are produced approximately isotropically and penetrate the head shielding in all directions.

Table 4-2 Relative yield of photoneutrons in semi-infinite thick targets as a function of the incident electron energy*

Target element	*Electron Energy (MeV)* 10	15	20	25
Al	0.0	0.0	0.0	0.03
Cu	0.0	0.0	0.11	0.25
Fe	0.0	0.0	0.07	0.17
Pb	0.0	0.25	0.70	0.93
W	0.0	0.25	0.70	1.00

*The data were calculated from values given in NCRP (1984) and normalized to one for tungsten at 25 MeV electron energy.

The energy spectrum of the photoneutrons is similar to a fission spectrum with a peak value near 2 MeV. Two groups of neutrons are produced in photoneutron reactions. One group has a Maxwellian energy distribution and is composed of evaporation neutrons. These constitute the majority of the photoneutrons. The second group is composed of direct neutrons, which are produced by a direct interaction between the photon and a neutron in the nucleus of the target atom. Direct neutrons make up approximately 15% of the photoneutrons, and they have a higher energy than the evaporation neutrons. Figure 4-3 shows a fission spectrum and a photoneutron spectrum. The direct neutrons appear as a small peak on the high-energy side of the photoneutron spectrum.

It should be pointed out that the neutron spectrum that exists in the accelerator room will be degraded in energy as a result of neutron

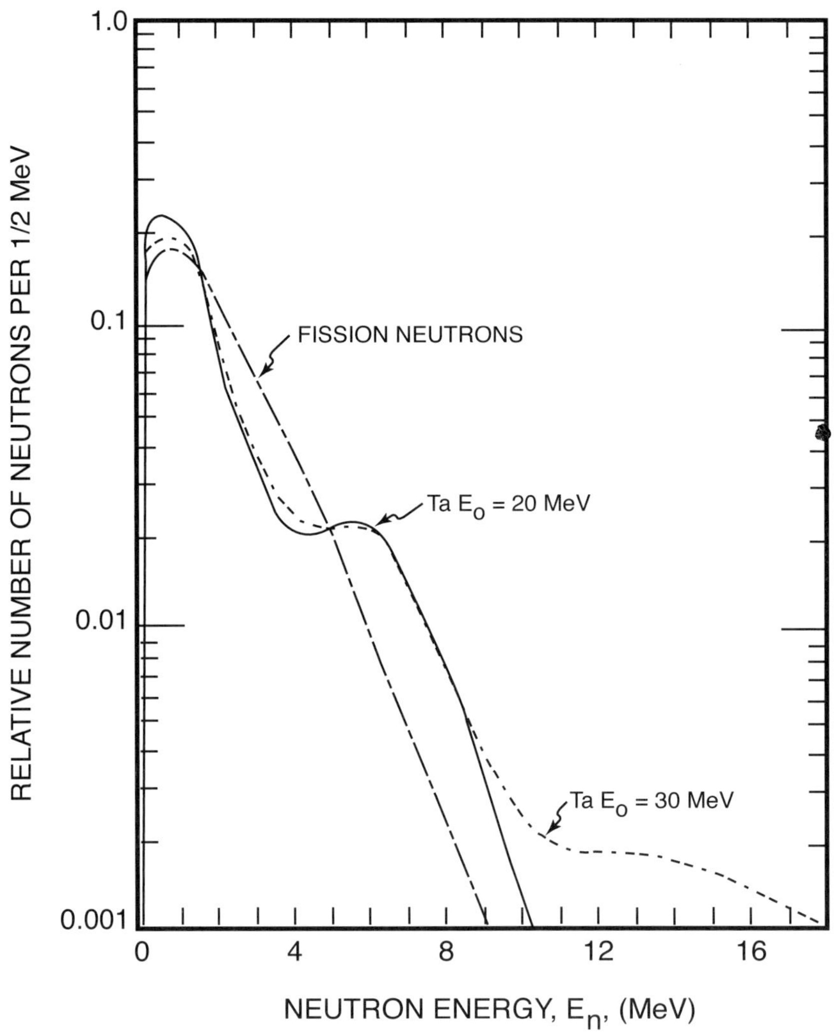

Figure 4-3. Typical photoneutron and fission energy spectrum. From NCRP 1964 with permission.

interactions in the accelerator structure and scattering from the concrete surfaces of the room. Very few of the photoneutrons are attenuated or lost in penetration through lead, and only a slight loss of about 15% occurs in an accelerator with tungsten head shielding. Techniques have been published (NCRP 1984) that can be used to evaluate the average neutron energy after the photoneutrons have penetrated different thicknesses of lead, steel, or tungsten. For example, the average neutron energy decreases from 2 MeV to 1.7 MeV after the neutrons pass through a typical head shield of 6.4 cm thickness of lead. The average energy of the room-scattered neutrons is obtained by multiplying the average energy of the neutrons emerging from the accelerator head by 0.24. This procedure gives an energy of 0.4 MeV for the room-scattered neutron component. In addition to the neutron energy groups mentioned above, there will be a thermal neutron energy group in the accelerator room.

As shown by equation 4-1, the total neutron fluence (n/cm^2) per unit dose of x-ray at the isocenter is given by the sum of the neutron components mentioned above.

$$\Phi = \Phi_{dir} + \Phi_{sc} + \Phi_{th} \qquad (4\text{-}1)$$

McCall et al. (1979) have found that the direct (dir) neutron fluence (n/cm^2) per unit dose of x-ray is given by

$$\Phi_{dir} = aQ/4\pi d^2 \qquad (4\text{-}2)$$

where a is the transmission factor for neutrons that penetrate the head shielding, d is the distance (cm) from the target to the point where the direct fluence is evaluated, and Q is the neutron source strength in neutrons emitted from the structure of the accelerator head per unit dose of x-ray delivered to the isocenter. The transmission factor (a) has a value of 1.0 for lead and 0.85 for tungsten shielding. It has been found (NCRP 1984) that the room scatter (Φ_{sc}) and the thermal neutron fluence (Φ_{th}) are each constant throughout the accelerator room. Equation 4-3 can be used to determine the thermal neutron fluence

$$\Phi_{th} = 1.26Q/S \qquad (4\text{-}3)$$

where S is the surface area of the treatment room in square centimeters. A similar equation can be used to establish the room-scattered neutron fluence.

$$\Phi_{sc} = 5.4aQ/S \qquad (4\text{-}4)$$

Combining equations 4-2, 4-3, and 4-4 to obtain the total neutron fluence per unit dose of x-ray at the isocenter gives equation 4-5.

$$\Phi = aQ/4\pi d^2 + 5.4aQ/S + 1.26Q/S \tag{4-5}$$

Values of the neutron source strength (Q) are available in the literature for most medical accelerators (McCall 1987, McGinley and Landry 1989, McGinley et al. 1993, and Fenn and McGinley 1995). Table 4-3 summarizes Q values for a number of modern accelerators.

Table 4-3 Neutron source strength for medical accelerators

Manufacturer	*Model*	*Stated MeV**	*Q (neutrons per Gy)*
Siemens	KD	20	0.92×10^{12}
Varian	1800	18	1.22
Varian	1800	15	0.76
Varian	1800	10	0.06
Philips	SL-25	22	2.37
Philips	SL-20	17	0.69
GE	Saturne 43	25	2.40
GE	Saturne 43	18	1.50
GE	Saturne 41	15	0.47
GE	Saturne 41	12	0.24

*Energy given by manufacturer.

The neutron source strengths measured by the author for the more recent Varian accelerator models (2100C/D and 2300C/D) are similar to the values given for the Varian 1800 series shown in Table 4-3. In chapter 5 the techniques used to evaluate the neutron fluence (presented in this chapter) will be used to determine the neutron dose equivalent at the maze entrance of the treatment room.

State Rules and Regulations for Head Leakage

Most state rules and regulations concerning medical accelerators require the radiation level due to neutrons and photons leaking through the head shielding to meet the requirements outlined below.

1. For operations producing the maximum leakage radiation, the absorbed dose due to neutrons and photons, at any point in a circular plane (patient plane or area) of two meters radius centered on and perpendicular to the central axis of the beam at the isocenter and outside the maximum beam size, shall not exceed 0.1% of the absorbed dose due to x-rays at the isocenter. Measurements excluding neutrons are averaged over an area up to 100 cm^2 size. Due to the size of typical neutron dosimeters the neutron dose is averaged over 200 cm^2. Figure 4-4 illustrates the location of the patient plane or area for a beam directed downward.

2. Points outside the patient area and at one meter from the path of the electron beam through the accelerator shall receive an absorbed dose due to photons that is ≤ 0.1% of the x-ray dose at the isocenter and ≤ 0.05% due to neutrons.

An interesting situation develops if the neutron absorbed dose is converted to dose equivalent using the recommended quality factor of 10 or 20 for fast neutrons. Making this conversion could result in a neutron leakage level as high as 0.01 or 0.02 Sv neutrons per Gy of x-ray at the isocenter. For a treatment dose of 70 Gy of x-ray, the total body

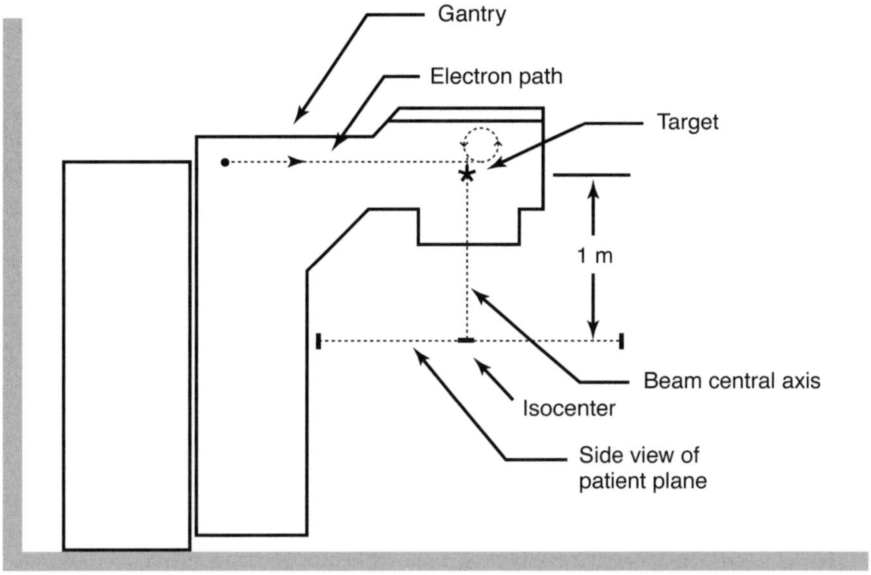

Figure 4-4. Side view of accelerator and the patient plane. The patient plane is a horizontal plane of 2 m radius centered on the beam central axis.

dose equivalent due to neutrons will be of the order of 0.7 to 1.4 Sv. Kliauga and Amols (1995) have estimated that a neutron leakage level of 2.3 mSv neutrons per Gy of x-ray would produce 500 malignancies per year in long-term radiotherapy survivors treated to 70 Gy tumor dose. Scaling this figure up to the state limits would give 2200 to 4300 new cancer cases per year. This is a gross overestimation because most medical accelerators operating above 15 MeV have neutron dose equivalent levels in the patient plane of approximately 1 to 2 mSv per Gy of x-ray at the isocenter.

Activation of Materials

An additional complication caused by photoneutron reactions from high-energy medical acceleratorsis that a number of materials found in the accelerator head become radioactive as a result of photon (γ,n) and neutron capture (n,γ) reactions in the target, flattening filter, and collimators. Technicians who enter the treatment room after the accelerator run has been terminated will be exposed to gamma radiation from the induced activity. Wedge filters and field defining blocks also become radioactive when placed in the beam, and the hands of the technician will be exposed to gamma and beta radiation. Table 4-4 lists some of the radioactive isotopes identified by Almen et al. (1991) in accelerators operated above 12 MeV.

Table 4-4 Radionuclides produced in medical accelerators

Reaction	*Mode of decay*	*Half-life*	*Photon energy (MeV)*
$^{27}Al(n,\gamma)^{28}Al$	β-	2.3 min	1.780
$^{63}Cu(\gamma,n)^{62}Cu$	β+	9.7 min	0.511
$^{55}Mn(n,\gamma)^{56}Mn$	β-	2.6 hr	0.847
$^{63}Cu(n,\gamma)^{64-}Cu$	β+/β-	12.7 hr	1.346
$^{65}Cu(\gamma,n)^{64}Cu$	β+/β-	12.7 hr	1.346
$^{186}W(n,\gamma)^{187}W$	β-	23.9 hr	0.479/0.686
$^{58}Ni(\gamma,n)^{57}Ni$	β+	36.0 hr	1.378/1.920

It is interesting to note that no radionuclides resulting from reactions with lead were detected by Almen et al. (1991). Near the accelerator the dose rate immediately after treatment is dominated by ^{28}Al and ^{62}Cu, and after one hour the longer-lived isotopes ^{187}W and ^{57}Ni produce the majority of the dose rate. It was found by Almen et al. (1991) that the annual dose received by the technician from induced activity was in the range 1.0 to 2.8 mGy for the trunk region of the body and 0.7 to 3.3 mGy for the hands. A workload of 240 work days per year and 3500 high-energy ports treated per year were used to estimate the annual dose.

The author measured the dose rate at the distal end of the collimator of a number of Varian 2100 and 2300 accelerators operated at 18 MeV and found an average level of 0.80 mGy per hour two minutes after the machine had been run for 30 minutes for testing purposes. Therefore, the maintenance engineer should not perform repair operations near the target and collimators within 40 minutes of a long test run. The nitrogen and oxygen that constitute the air in the treatment room become slightly radioactive due to (γ,n) reactions. Air activation is discussed in chapter 7.

Materials for Neutron Shielding

Fast neutrons produced by medical accelerators operating above 10 MeV are efficiently attenuated by materials with a high hydrogen content. Concrete, which is commonly used for photon shielding, contains a relatively high hydrogen content (as shown in Table 4-5). The photoneutrons from medical accelerators have a TVL of 21 cm in concrete, and the primary x-ray beam has a TVL of approximately 44 cm in concrete. This difference in TVL values for neutrons versus photons means that a concrete shield that produces adequate attenuation of the x-ray beam will provide more than sufficient attenuation of the photoneutrons. Fast neutrons are moderated or reduced in energy by elastic scattering from hydrogen and, after a number of collisions, become slow neutrons. Low-energy neutrons undergo capture reactions with many materials, and penetrating capture gamma rays are emitted. In concrete the capture gamma ray spectrum extends to above 8.0 MeV, and the average energy is 3.6 MeV. Capture of slow neutrons by hydrogen in concrete results in a pronounced peak in the photon spectrum at 2.21 MeV.

A number of materials, such as boron and cadmium, have large cross sections for slow neutron capture, and a few millimeters of the materials will absorb almost all of the neutrons. Boron can be incorporated into polyethylene, which has a high hydrogen content, to form an efficient neutron shield. Slow neutron capture in the boron results in the production of a relatively low-energy gamma ray (0.473 MeV). Therefore, polyethylene with a boron content of 5% by weight is commonly used in neutron-shielded doors for treatment rooms. The transmission of capture gamma rays through polyethylene cannot be represented by a simple exponential function, so a tenth value thickness is not given in Table 4-5. However, O'Brien et al. (1985) have published graphical data showing the attenuation of concrete capture gamma rays by polyethylene.

Table 4-5 Properties of shielding materials

Material	*Hydrogen content (atoms per cm³)*	*TVL fast neutrons (cm)*	*TVL slow neutrons (cm)*	*TVL capture gammas (cm)*	*Neutron activation*
concrete	0.8 to 2.4 $\times 10^{22}$	21.0*	34.0	45.0	low
polyethylene	8×10^{22}	4.5†	77.0	—	very low
(5%B)	—	—	1.27	—	very low
steel	—	—	10.7	13.5	medium
lead	—	—	410	6.1	low

*head leakage neutrons
†maze neutrons

Problems

1. Determine the neutron fluence at the inner maze entrance per cGy of x-ray delivered to the isocenter for the treatment room described in chapter 2, problem 7. Assume that the accelerator is operated at 18 MeV and is constructed of lead. Note that McGinley and Landry (1989) found that the surface area (S) should be calculated for a room with primary barriers that project into the room using the average width, length, and height of the room.

2. What fraction of the neutron fluence at the inner maze entrance is due to each of the following components?
   a. direct neutrons
   b. room scattered neutrons
   c. thermal neutrons

3. Evaluate the neutron fluence per cGy of x-ray at a point in the patient plane (1 m from the isocenter in a horizontal direction with the beam directed vertically down).

4. Determine for lead the isotopes produced by the (γ,n) and (n,γ) reaction. Which are radioactive and what is the half-life of each?

5

Mazes and Doors for High-Energy Rooms

Neutron Shielding

Most medical accelerators operating above 10 MeV use a maze with a door shielded for neutrons and photons at the outer maze entrance. A typical door consists of a steel case 0.635 cm thick containing 10.2 cm of borated polyethylene (5% B by weight) and a 1.27 cm lead slab. The polyethylene is used to moderate the fast and intermediate energy neutrons, which then react with the boron and produce a 0.473 MeV photon. The lead is placed after the polyethylene, where it will attenuate the photons produced in the boron and any capture gamma rays generated in the maze by neutron capture in the concrete walls, ceiling, and floor.

The evaluation of the neutron dose equivalent at the outer maze entrance is carried out using the method developed by Kersey (1979). This technique has been evaluated by McGinley and Butker (1991) for a number of treatment facilities and for a variety of accelerator models produced by several manufacturers. It was determined that the ratio of the neutron dose equivalent calculated by use of Kersey's method divided by the measured neutron level varied from 0.82 to 2.3 for the 13 accelerator facilities investigated in the study.

In use of Kersey's technique the effective neutron source position is taken to be the isocenter of the accelerator, and the neutron dose equivalent (H) at the entrance to the maze per unit dose of x-ray at the isocenter is given by the equation shown below.

$$H = (H_0)(T/T_0)(d_0/d_1)^2 10^{-d_2/5} \qquad (5\text{-}1)$$

where H_0 is the neutron dose equivalent at a distance d_0 from the target. Values of H_0 that have been measured by the author for a number of medical accelerators are shown in Table 5-1. The neutron head leakage (H_0) is made up of the dose equivalent due to direct, room scatter, and thermal neutrons; the last two components change with the treatment room surface area. For a small room, the scattered and thermal neutron levels are greater than those for a large room.

Table 5-1 Neutron dose equivalent H_0 at 1.41 m from the target per unit dose of x-ray at the isocenter (mSv n/Gy X)

Accelerator manufacturer	*Model*	*Stated (MeV)*	*Beam MV**	*H_0 (mSv n/Gy x)*	*Reference*
Varian	1800	18	16.8	1.02 - 1.60	unpublished
	1800	15	U†	0.79 - 1.30	"
	1800	10	U†	0.04	"
Siemens	KD	20	16.5	1.10 - 1.24	McGinley 1988
	MD	15	U†	0.17	unpublished
Philips	SL-25	25	22.0	2.00	McGinley et al. 1993
	SL-20	20	17.0	0.44	"
GE Saturne	43	25	18.5	1.38	Fenn and McGinley 1995
	43	18	14.0	0.55	"
	41	15	12.5	0.32	"
	41	12	11.2	0.09	"

*Based on AAPM TG-21 protocol (AAPM 1983).
†Unknown.

T/T_0 is the ratio of the outer maze area to the inner maze entrance area. Distance d_1 (shown in figure 5-1) is the distance in meters from the isocenter to the point on the maze center line from which the isocenter is just visible. For a maze with one bend, d_2 is the distance

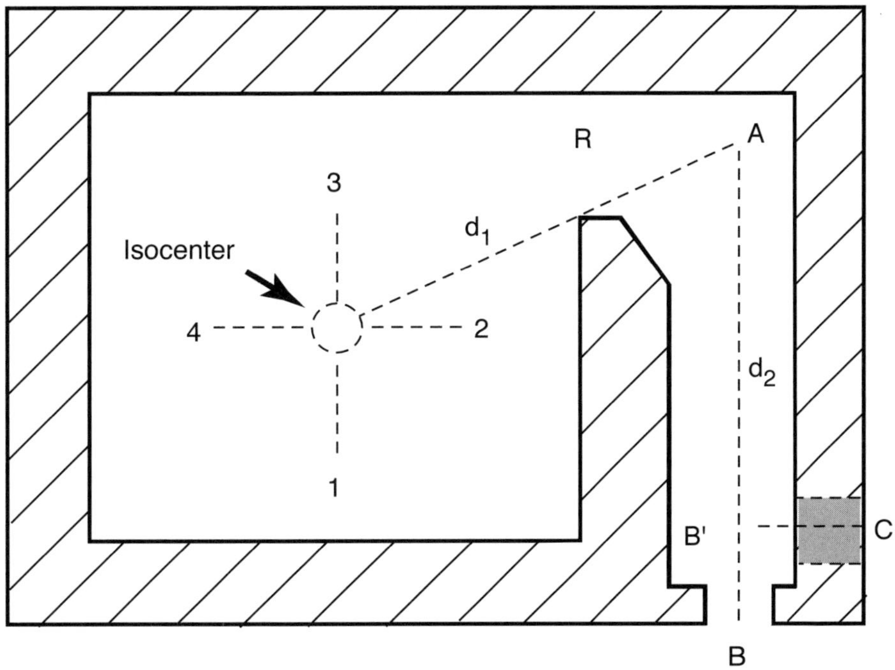

Figure 5-1 Floor plan for accelerator room and maze

from A to B of figure 5-1. In the case of a maze with two bends, d_2 is the distance from A to B′ plus B′ length to C of figure 5-1. Note that the maze has a tenth value distance (TVD) of 5 m for the attenuation of neutrons. McGinley and Butker (1991) found that the TVD for maze neutrons was approximately 16% less than 5 m. Therefore, 5 m is a conservative value to use for the neutron TVD when the dose equivalent is determined at the maze outer entrance. It was also discovered that a second turn in the maze reduced the neutron level by a factor of about three as compared with the value obtained by Kersey's equation.

For a maze with two bends, equation 5-1 is modified as shown below to account for the second turn.

$$H = H_0\,(T/T_0)\,(d_0/d_1)^2(10^{-d_2/5})(10^{-d_3/5})(1/3) \qquad (5\text{-}2)$$

Distance d_3 is equivalent to the distance between points B′ and C of figure 5-1 expressed in meters.

The neutron level at the maze entrance varies with the collimator setting, with the maximum value obtained by closing the collimators. The maximum increase in the neutron dose at the outer maze entrance is on the order of 15% when the collimator size is reduced from 40 × 40 cm^2 to 0 × 0 cm^2. The neutron field is also a function of the gantry angle and location of the target rotational plane in the treatment room. For example, McGinley and Butker (1991) reported that the neutron level at the treatment room door was at a maximum level when the target rotational plane was aligned along the line marked 1-3 of figure 5-1 and the gantry angle was set to give a horizontal beam directed from point 3 to point 1. This alignment places the neutron source (the target) closer to the inner maze entrance than other positions of the gantry and the target rotational plane. Table 5-2 shows the variation in the relative neutron and photon dose equivalent at the outer maze door based on the average of measurements made at 15 treatment rooms. All data in Table 5-2 have been normalized to one for the vertical down beam direction, and the target rotational plane for each room was along line 1–3 of figure 5-1.

Table 5-2 Relative neutron and photon dose equivalent at the outer maze entrance as a function of beam direction.* Beam direction based on Figure 5-1.

Stated energy (MeV)	*Relative neutron dose equivalent*				*Relative photon dose equivalent*			
	1 to 3	3 to 1	up	down	1 to 3	3 to 1	up	down
18	0.68	1.17	0.74	1.00	0.75	1.13	0.89	1.00
15	0.83	1.20	1.09	1.00	0.88	1.25	0.90	1.00

*All data have been normalized to 1.00 for the down beam direction.

It has been found by McGinley et al. (1995c) that a plot of the neutron dose equivalent as a function of the distance d_2 along the maze centerline could be resolved into the sum of two exponential functions as shown by the equation below.

$$H = H_1 10^{-d_2/TVDN1} + H_2 10^{-d_2/TVDN2} \quad (5\text{-}3)$$

The smaller TVDN is designated TVDN1 and the larger TVDN2. The value of TVDN2 was obtained from a semilog plot of the dose equivalent versus the distance from point A of figure 5-1. The curve, which is a straight line for values of d_2 greater than 3 m, was extrapolated to the point where d_2 was zero, the value of H_2 was read from the curve, and the slope of the line was used to evaluate TVDN2. A subtraction of the extrapolated curve from the measured neutron dose equivalent curve yields a second straight line from which the value of TVDN1 and H_1 can be obtained. Figure 5-2, which is for photons, is similar in shape to the semilog plot of the neutron dose equivalent along the

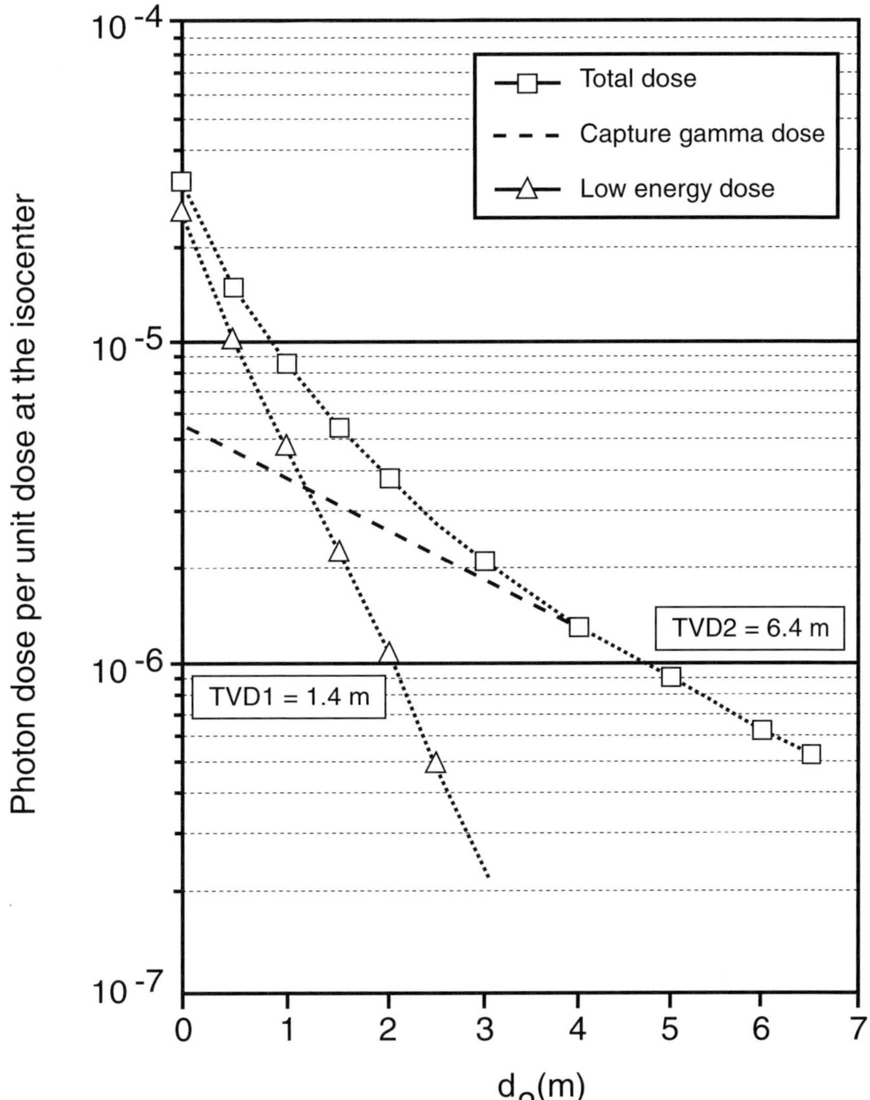

Figure 5-2. Photon dose along the maze center line per unit dose of 18 MV x-ray at the isocenter. From McGinley et al. 1995b with permission.

maze center line. The uncertainty of the TVDN values is ± 0.2 m. The larger TVDN has a value of approximately 5.0 m, which is in good agreement with Kersey's (Kersey 1979) measurements, and the smaller TVDN is approximately 1.7 m. Therefore, the neutron dose equivalent falls off faster in the first three meters of maze length than indicated by Kersey's technique.

Based on the neutron level at the outer maze entrance, the amount of borated polyethylene needed for radiation protection can be determined using the tenth value layer in polyethylene given in NCRP Report No. 79 (NCRP 1984) as function of neutron energy. The average neutron energy at the maze entrance has been reported to be approximately 100 keV, and the corresponding TVL in polyethylene is 4.5 cm (NCRP 1984).

Capture Gamma Ray Shielding

Most accelerator doors have a lead component that is designed to attenuate the x-rays scattered from the treatment room into the maze. However, an additional photon component with high energy will be present at the treatment room door due to neutron capture in the materials used to construct the maze. Tochlin and LaRiviere (1979) reported that the average energy of capture gamma rays from concrete is 3.6 MeV. A method for estimating the photon dose at the treatment room door has been devised by McGinley et al. (1995b) based on a technique similar to the one described above in which the neutron dose equivalent is resolved into two exponential functions. Figure 5-2 shows the photon dose distribution along the maze center line and the two exponential components. The capture gamma dose (D) at the maze entrance per dose of x-ray at the isocenter is given by the equation shown below.

$$D = K\Phi_{total} 10^{-d_2/TVD2} \tag{5-4}$$

where K is the ratio of the capture gamma dose to the total neutron fluence at point A of figure 5-1. Based on experimental data, an average value of 0.77×10^{-12} cm^2 Gy was found for K. The tenth value distance, TVD2, is approximately 6.2 m for 16.2 to 22 MV x-ray beams. The total neutron fluence (cm^{-2}) at point A per unit dose (Gy) of x-ray at the isocenter is represented by Φ_{total}. For mazes where the distance from A to B of figure 5-1 is greater than 3 m, the photon field is dominated by capture gamma rays and the x-ray scatter component can be ignored. In fact, the photon dose outside the maze door changes only slightly when the collimator of the accelerator is adjusted from maximum size to the closed position. This behavior is not unexpected if the photon field at the outer maze entrance is due primarily to capture gamma rays formed in the maze by neutron interactions.

It has been observed that the total neutron fluence at the inner maze entrance per unit dose of x-ray at the isocenter can be evaluated by use of the equation given below (NCRP 1984 and McCall et al. 1979).

$$\Phi_{total} = Qa/4\pi d_1^2 + 5.4aQ/S + 1.26Q/S \qquad (5\text{-}5)$$

Where a is the transmission factor for neutrons that penetrate the head shielding, d_1 is the distance in centimeters from the isocenter to point A of figure 5-1, Q is the neutron source strength in neutrons emitted from the accelerator head per unit dose of x-ray at the isocenter, and S is the surface area of the treatment room in square centimeters. The transmission factor has a value of 1.0 for lead and 0.85 for tungsten head shielding. Values of the neutron source strength (Q) are available in the literature for most medical accelerators (McCall 1987, McGinley and Landry 1989, McGinley 1988, and McGinley et al. 1993), and typical values are given in Table 4-3. After the capture gamma ray dose level at the outer maze entrance has been calculated, the thickness of lead needed in the treatment room door can be determined using a TVL of 6.1 cm (NCRP 1984).

The procedure outlined above results in a heavy and expensive door that must be equipped with a motorized opener. It has been suggested (NCRP 1984) that by keeping the neutrons out of the maze, the door shielding can be reduced in thickness or eliminated completely. McGinley et al. (1995c) investigated three techniques, outlined below, to prevent neutrons from leaving the treatment room and entering the maze:

a. Reduce the opening at the inner maze entrance
b. Add a lightweight door containing a thermal neutron absorber at the inner maze entrance
c. Place a polyethylene (5% boron) door at the inner maze entrance

Table 5-3 indicates the dose equivalent rate at the outer maze entrance for a conventional maze and for mazes using the above techniques. Each maze has a length d_2 of 6.5 m, and the accelerators were operated at an x-ray dose rate of 6.67 cGy per second at the isocenter. The nominal megavoltage of each accelerator was 18 MV.

Table 5-3 Radiation dose equivalent rate due to capture gamma rays and neutrons at the outer maze entrance*

Type of maze and door	*Capture gamma dose equivalent rate (nSv s^{-1})*	*Neutron dose equivalent rate (nSv s^{-1})*	*Total N+g rate (nSv s^{-1})*
Conventional	38.8	116.3	155.1
a. Reduced inner opening	17.5	38.8	56.3
b. Inner boron door	12.7	31.9	44.6
c. Inner poly. door	6.9	10.2	17.1

* The maze length is 6.5 m and the dose rate at isocenter is 6.67 cGy/s.

In approach a, the inner maze opening was reduced in area using concrete 45.7 cm thick surrounding the opening, which was 1.22 × 2.13 m^2 in size. A panel 7 mm thick containing 8.9% boron by weight was employed for approach b, and a 5 cm thick polyethylene (5% boron) door was used for technique c. Method c produced the largest reduction in total dose equivalent, and as can be seen from Table 5-4, an outer maze door is not required for a maze with d_2 equal to 6.5 m and an accelerator workload of 500 Gy in seven days.

Table 5-4 Total radiation dose equivalent at the outer maze entrance for a workload of 500 Gy per week and a maze length of 6.5 m

Facility	*Photon dose equivalent per week (cSv)*	*Neutron dose equivalent per week (cSv)*	*Total dose equivalent per week (cSv)*
Conventional	0.0250	0.0710	0.0960
No door (a)	0.0105	0.0246	0.0351
Boron door (b)	0.0077	0.0187	0.0264
Poly. door (c)	0.0041	0.0058	0.0099

All other maze arrangements described above require an outer shielded door. Comparing the photon dose equivalent for the room with the boron panel with the room with no door, one sees that the capture gamma ray dose at the outer maze entrance is reduced by only 33% by the door. This indicates that the majority of the capture gamma rays are not produced by the slow neutrons that enter the maze from the treatment room but are produced by intermediate energy and fast neutrons that enter the maze and become thermalized.

Direct Shielded Doors

A direct shielded door located in a secondary wall can be used to enter the treatment room in place of a maze (McGinley 1993a). With this arrangement the floor space of the facility and the walking distance for the technician and patient can be reduced. A typical direct shielded or sliding door is shown in figure 5-3. The photon flux from room scatter and head leakage is attenuated by a 5.08 cm thick lead slab located on the treatment room side of the door. Next is a 27 cm thick polyethylene (5% by weight boron) layer that attenuates photoneutrons. This is followed by 10.2 cm of lead, which shields from the photons produced in the polyethylene by neutron reactions and from photons leaking through the first lead layer. The inner and outer door faces are fabricated from 0.63 cm steel, and 2.54 cm steel covers the sides, top, and bottom of the door. The door provides three TVL of photon shielding and 2.1 TVL of neutron shielding. Note that the door overlaps the opening in the secondary wall by 12.7 cm at the sides and top; there is a 2.54 cm gap between the wall and the inner door face on the left side of the door as shown in figure 5-3. The gap on the right side is reduced to 1.27 cm by a layer of polyethylene to prevent neutrons from streaming out of the room. A polyethylene and lead "stop post" is on the left side of the door to reduce the photon and neutron dose level.

The door moves on rollers located on the bottom and top of the door, and the total mass of the door is approximately 7260 kg. Motion detectors will stop the movement of the door if anyone approaches within 0.91 m. The door is opened and closed by a hydraulic ram and has an opening and closing time of 10 s. It has a backup air drive to be used in case of a loss of electricity. Two people can open the door manually by releasing a locking pin in the hydraulic drive.

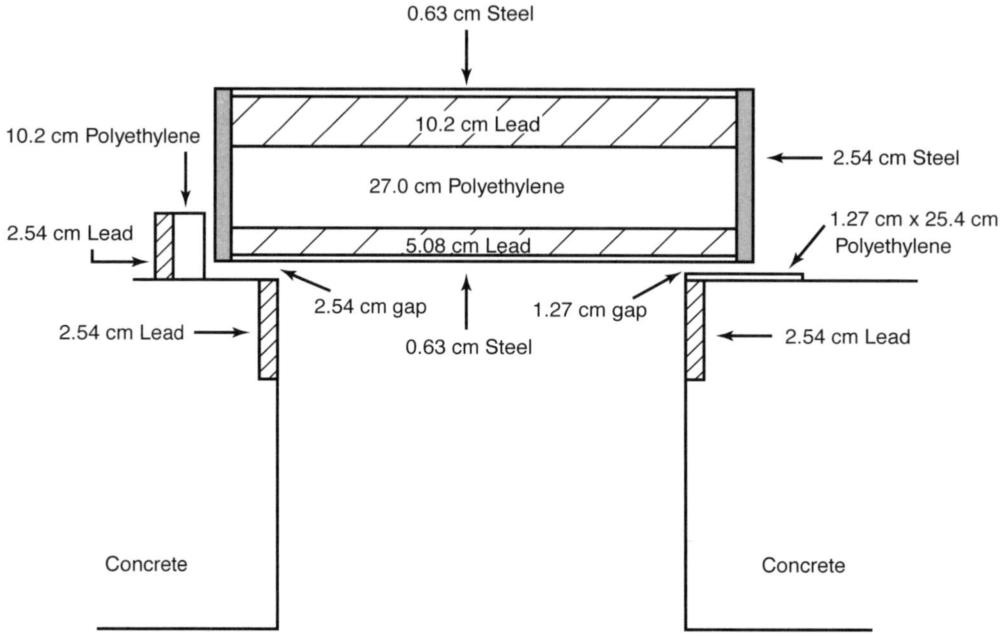

Figure 5-3. Direct shielded door for an 18 MeV accelerator

Figure 5-4 shows the floor plan of a room with a direct shielded door similar to that of figure 5-3. The room contains a Varian 2100C that operates in the 18 MV x-ray mode. An opening 122 cm long and 20 cm high for the heating, ventilation, and air conditioning (HVAC) system exists at ceiling level in the secondary wall. This opening is shielded with 5.08 cm of polyethylene and 2.54 cm of lead. A better system for the HVAC penetration would be to locate the HVAC duct under the floor slab and then bring it into the room through a floor opening.

The results of a radiation survey of the door and HVAC opening with the accelerator operated at 6.67 cGy/s at the isocenter are given in Table 5-5. Measurements were made with the collimator fully open (0.4×0.4 m^2) and closed, and a scattering phantom was located in the beam for all measurements. The maximum photon dose equivalent outside the room occurred when the collimator was opened to the maximum size, and the photon dose fell by 50% or less when the collimator was closed. On the other hand, the neutron dose equivalent was at a maximum with the collimators closed, and a 15% decrease was produced by opening the collimator.

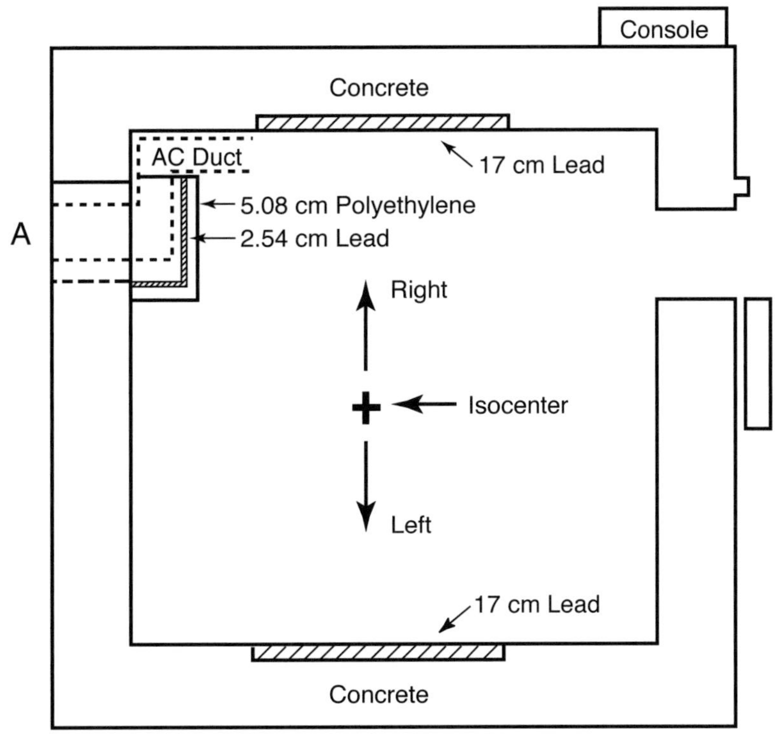

Figure 5-4. Floor plan for a treatment room with a direct shielded door

The expected radiation levels at the four points listed in Table 5-5 for one hour of operation, seven consecutive days, and one year of operation are given in Table 5-6. A workload of 20 Gy in any one hour of operation and 500 Gy in any seven days for the 18 MV x-ray beam was assumed for the accelerator. A use factor (U) of 1/4 and an occupancy factor (T) of one were used to determine the dose equivalent in seven days and for one year, and both T and U were made one for the one hour dose equivalent evaluation.

Based on Table 5-6 it can be seen that the radiation levels at the facility are well below the limits of 5×10^4 μSv per year for radiation workers. The radiation levels are also less than the limit of 1×10^3 μSv per year for the general public, except at the door frame. The shielding also meets the requirement that the dose equivalent be less than 20 μSv in any one hour for an unrestricted area.

Table 5-5 Maximum dose equivalent rates at the sliding door, console, and gonad levels below the HVAC penetration*

Beam direction	*Location*	*Dose equivalent rate* Neutron ($nSv\ s^{-1}$)	Photon ($nSv\ s^{-1}$)	Total (N+X) ($nSv\ s^{-1}$)
Down	door face	0.94	0.89	1.83
	door frame	1.64	3.31	4.95
	below HVAC	< 0.20	1.09	< 1.29
	console	< 0.20	0.33	< 0.53
Up	door face	1.06	0.64	1.70
	door frame	1.39	3.06	4.45
	below HVAC	< 0.20	1.09	< 1.29
	console	< 0.20	0.33	< 0.53
Right	door face	2.86	0.67	3.53
	door frame	2.06	3.31	5.37
	below HVAC	< 0.20	1.04	< 1.24
	console	< 0.20	0.33	< 0.53
Left	door face	1.56	0.64	2.20
	door frame	2.61	3.28	5.89
	below HVAC	< 0.20	3.04	< 3.24
	console	< 0.20	0.36	< 0.56

*The accelerator operating at 6.67 $cGy\ s^{-1}$ at the isocenter for the 18 MV x-ray mode

Table 5-6 Maximum total dose equivalent expected in any one hour of operation, in seven consecutive days, and in one year

Location	*Total dose equivalent (N + X)* One hour (m Sv)	Seven days (m Sv)	Annual (m Sv)
Door face	1.06	17.4	870
Door frame	1.77	38.7	1930
Below HVAC	0.97	9.5	475
Console	< 0.17	< 4.0	< 200

Example Calculations

1. Evaluate the capture gamma photon dose at the outer maze entrance of a room with the following dimensions.
   $d_1 = 6.34$ m $d_2 = 6.55$ m surface area (S) $= 1.96 \times 10^6$ cm^2
   neutron source strength (Q) $= 2 \times 10^{10}$ n/cGy at the isocenter

a. First determine Φ_{total}

$$\Phi_{total} = Q/4\pi d_1^2 + 6.66Q/S \qquad a = 1 \text{ (lead head)}$$

$$\Phi_{total} = 2 \times 10^{10}/4(\pi)(634^2) + 6.66(2 \times 10^{10})/1.96 \times 10^6$$

$$\Phi_{total} = 7.20 \times 10^4 \text{ n/cm}^2\text{/cGy X at the isocenter}$$

b. Now calculate the gamma dose based on Φ_{total}

$$D = K(\Phi_{total})10^{-d_2/TVD2}$$

$$D = 0.77 \times 10^{-10}(7.20 \times 10^4)(10^{-6.55/6.2})$$

$$D = 0.49 \times 10^{-6} \text{cGy/cGy at the isocenter}$$

c. Gamma dose per week
   D(week) $= D \times 50{,}000$ cGy/wk $= 0.025$ cGy/wk $= 25$ mrem γ/wk

2. Use Kersey's method to determine the neutron dose equivalent at the outer maze entrance of problem 1 for one week of operation. Assume that the maze area ratio is 1.0 and that the neutron leakage at 1.41 m from the target is 1.2 mrem n/cGy X at the isocenter.

$$H = W \times H_0 \times (1.41/d_1)^2 \times 10^{-d_2/5}$$

$$H = 50{,}000(1.2)(1.41/6.34)^2 \times (10^{-6.55/5})$$

$$H = 145 \text{ mrem n/wk}$$

3. Determine the thickness of lead and polyethylene needed in the treatment room door.
a. polyethylene (TVLN = 4.5 cm for maze neutrons)

To reduce the dose equivalent to the ALARA level of 10 mrem/wk we will assume that half is neutron and half capture gamma rays.

$$5/145 = 10^{-s/4.5} \text{ and } s = 6.6 \text{ cm poly.}$$

b. To reduce the capture gamma dose equivalent to 5 mrem/wk we need the following thickness of lead.

$$5/25 = 10^{-s/6.1} \quad s = 4.26 \text{ cm lead}$$

Note that most doors use more polyethylene and less lead for example, 4″ of polyethylene plus a 1/4″ steel case. The neutron dose equivalent will now be:

$$H = 145 \times 10^{-4 \times 2.54/4.5} = 0.80 \text{ mrem/wk.}$$

We will now need to reduce the capture gamma dose equivalent to 10 - 0.80 = 9.20 mrem/wk for ALARA. The lead thickness needed is given by $9.20/25 = 10^{-s/6.1}$ and $s = 2.6$ cm. This can be reduced to 2.0 cm of lead due to the steel case.

One could reduce the lead thickness further because of the attenuation of the capture gamma rays in the 4″ of polyethylene. Based on the average energy of the capture gamma rays from concrete, the transmission through the polyethylene will be approximately 70%. Therefore, the lead layer can be reduced by 0.95 cm ($0.70 = 10^{-s/6.1}$ and $s = 0.95$ cm lead equivalent). A lead thickness of 2.0 - 0.95 = 1.05 cm will be used in the door. The gamma rays generated in the polyethylene (5% by weight B) by the $^{10}B(n,\gamma)$ reaction are of 0.473 MeV energy, and only 8% of the photons will be transmitted through the 1.05 cm of lead. Figure 5-5 shows the design of the maze door.

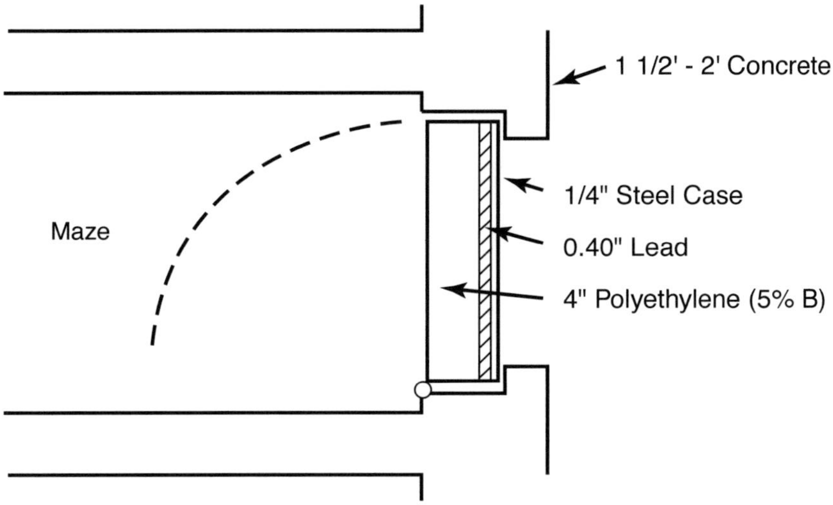

Figure 5-5. Neutron and photon shielded door for the outer maze entrance

Problems

1. Determine the neutron and photon dose equivalent per week at the outer maze entrance of the treatment room described in problem 7, chapter 2. The accelerator is operated at 18 MeV, and the maze area ratio is one. Assume a lead head machine and a workload of 50,000 cGy per week at the isocenter.
2. Design a door for the maze described in problem 1.
3. Repeat problem 1 for the case where the door is located at the end of the maze on the console wall (2 turn maze) and the area ratio for the maze is 1/2. Is a shielded door needed for the room?
4. a. Determine the tenth value layer (TVL) in lead for the capture gamma rays produced in concrete.
   b. Repeat part a for the gamma photons from the $^{10}B(n, \gamma)$ reaction.

6

Metal and Concrete Shields

Primary Barriers Containing Metal

Lead and steel are occasionally used in the construction of primary barriers for treatment rooms containing high-energy accelerators operating above 10 MeV. In general, lead or steel is used with concrete for shielding when there is limited space for the barrier or when a low-energy accelerator room is upgraded to house a high-energy accelerator. A radiological health hazard may be created when these metals are used in primary barriers because of the production of photoneutrons when the beam is aimed at the shield. Steel has a photoneutron cross section that is 10 times less than that of lead and presents a less significant source of neutrons. McGinley et al. (1988) and McGinley (1992a, and 1992b) have investigated the use of metals in primary shields, and the following is a summary of these studies.

Figure 6-1 illustrates a situation that can occur outside a primary barrier when the beam is incident on the shield. The direct neutrons leaking from the accelerator head are reduced in intensity by inverse square fall-off and attenuation in the concrete portion of the shield. If the concrete part of the shield is at least a few feet thick, the machine neutrons are reduced to a low level and can be ignored. However, the photon beam will produce photoneutrons in the lead shield that in

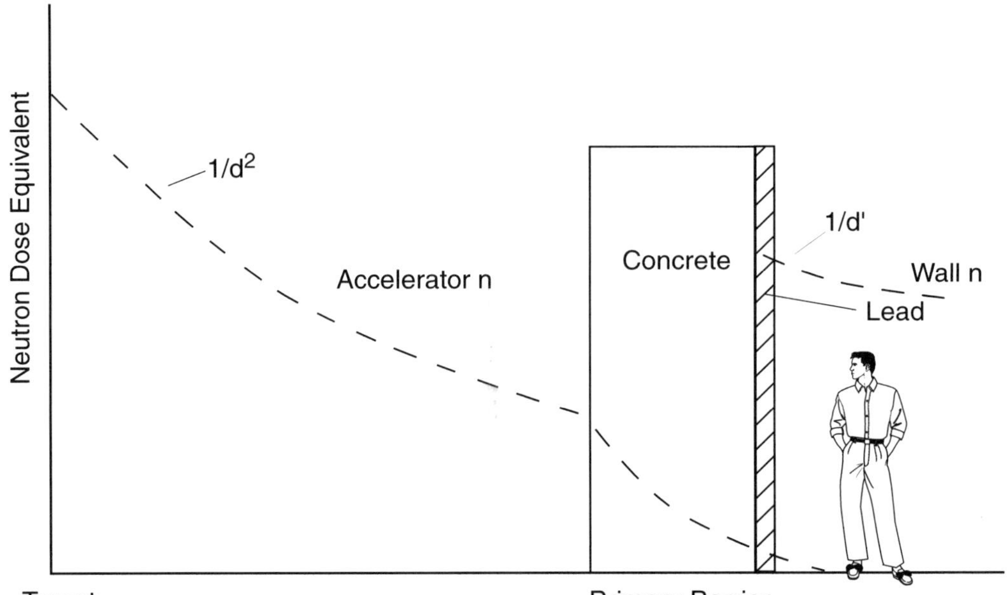

Figure 6-1. Accelerator and wall neutrons

this case are not attenuated by concrete while emerging from the shield. The fall-off of neutron intensity from the lead with distance is at a lower rate than the fall-off of machine neutrons because the lead layer acts as a large volume source. Instead of following the inverse square law, the neutrons produced in the lead slab fall off approximately at the inverse of the distance from the wall.

The location and thickness of the metal layer in a composite concrete and metal barrier are very important. As can be seen from figure 6-2, all of the shields produce about the same photon attenuation. However, the neutron dose equivalent varies by a factor of more than 500 depending on the location and thickness of the lead slab. In all three cases shown in figure 6-2, the x-ray dose rate at the isocenter was 6.67 cGy s^{-1} and the beam was aimed at the primary barrier. Lead is a very poor neutron attenuator, and it also acts as a source of neutrons when the beam strikes it. Concrete is a good neutron attenuator, and if lead is substituted for part of the concrete in a shield, the neutron transmission is increased. In addition, the metal acts as a source of neutrons when the beam impinges on the shield. If there is insufficient concrete beyond the metal, the neutrons produced in the lead will irradiate personnel outside the barrier.

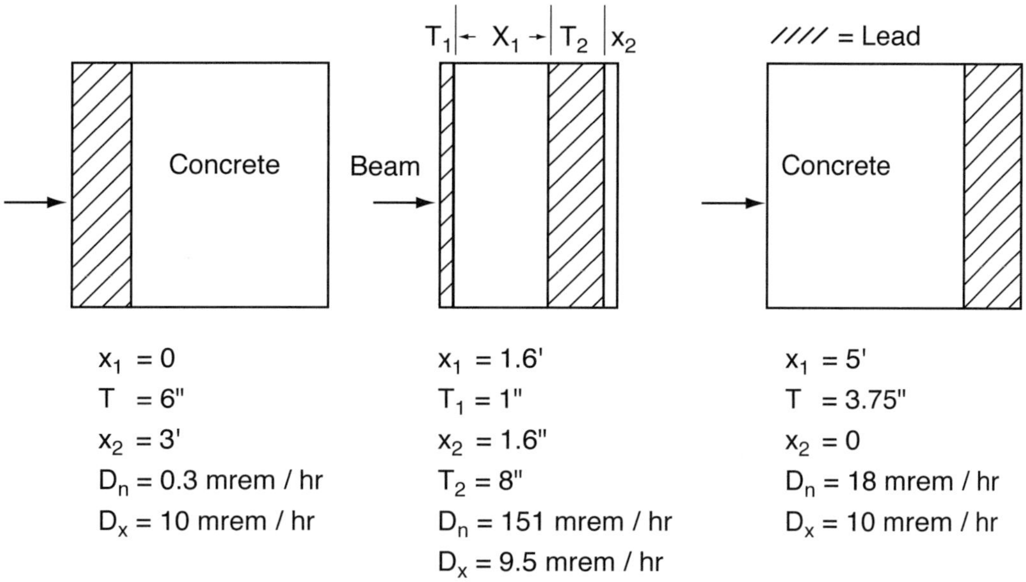

Figure 6-2. Neutron and photon dose equivalent rate outside primary shield for 40 x 40 cm^2 beam and 400 cGy/min dose rate at isocenter. The megavoltage of the beam is 18 MV.

McGinley (1992a) has shown that the neutron dose equivalent outside a concrete barrier that contains lead or steel is given by equation 6-1. This empirical equation was established for situations in which the collimator is open to maximum size.

$$H = \frac{D_X PB}{(T/2 + X_2 + 0.305)} 10^{-X_1/TVLX}\, 10^{-X_2/TVLN} \qquad (6\text{-}1)$$

where

- H = neutron dose equivalent rate ($\mu Sv\ s^{-1}$)
- D = x-ray dose rate at the isocenter ($cGy\ s^{-1}$)
- X_1 = thickness of first concrete slab (m)
- X_2 = thickness of final layer of concrete (m)
- T = thickness of metal slab (m)
- P = neutron production rate (μSv neutron cGy^{-1} x-ray m^{-2} beam area)

B = maximum beam area at isocenter (m^2)

TVLX = tenth value layer in concrete for primary x-rays (m)

TVLN = tenth value layer in concrete for photoneutrons (m)

0.305m = distance from outer surface of barrier to point protected.

Accelerators operating at 18 MeV had maximum neutron production values (P) of 19 and 1.7 μSv neutron per cGy x-ray m^2 beam area for lead and steel, respectively. When the accelerator is operated at 15 MeV, P decreases by a factor of 5.4 for lead.

Based on equation 6-1, the maximum neutron dose equivalent is produced when lead is placed on the outside of the concrete ($X_2 = 0$) and the lead has a large thickness. Figure 6-3 illustrates this principle

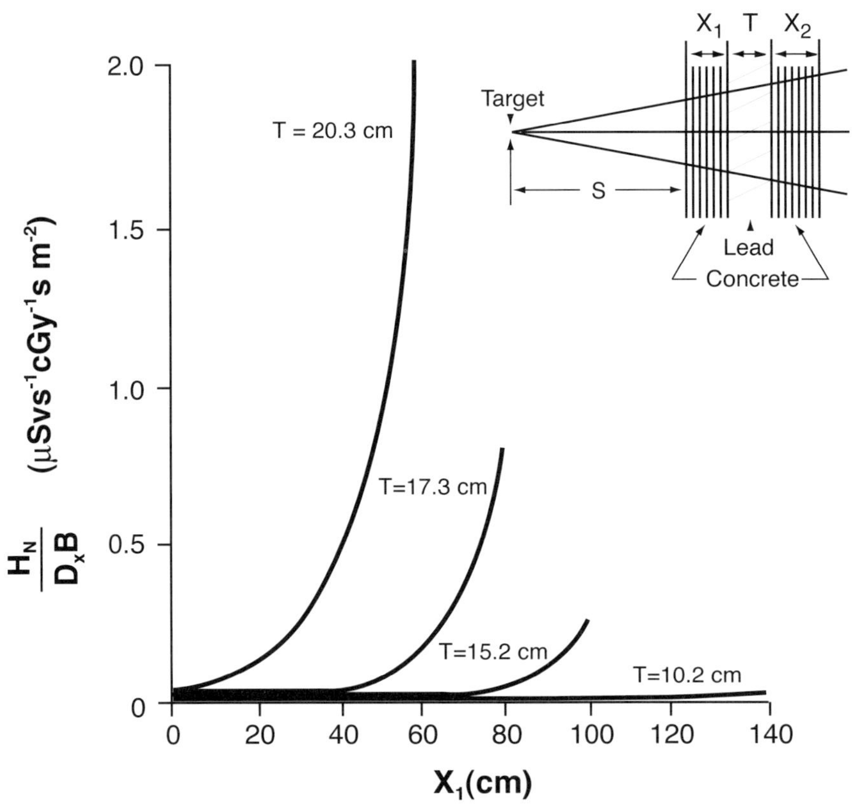

Figure 6-3. Neutron dose equivalent rate normalized to unit x-ray dose rate at isocenter and unit beam area versus position of lead slab in shield. The barrier is equivalent to 5 TVL for 18 MV x-ray. From McGinley (1993a) with permission.

for a barrier that contains 5 TVL of shielding material for an 18 MV x-ray. Each curve is for a fixed lead thickness (T) with the position of the lead slab varying from inside the room to the outside. A TVLN of 0.21 m of concrete was used for photoneutrons produced in the lead portion of the shield, and a TVLX of 0.445 m for the primary 18 MV beam in concrete. As can be seen, the neutron dose equivalent rate increases as more concrete is replaced by lead and as the lead portion of the shield is placed closer to the outside surface of the shield (x_1 increasing). Note that in all cases the shield is equivalent to 5 TVL for the photon beam.

To summarize, if a lead slab is to be used in a primary barrier it should be placed on the inside of the treatment room and at least 2.5' of concrete should be installed beyond the lead to provide adequate neutron shielding. Replacing the lead with steel will lower the neutron production in the metal by a factor of about 10.

Example Calculation

1. Determine the neutron dose equivalent rate outside the primary shield shown in figure 6-4 (next page). The accelerator is operated at 18 MeV, the dose rate at the isocenter is 400 cGy/min, and the beam size is 40×40 cm^2.

   Using equation 6-1 we have:

$$H = \frac{(6.67)(19)(0.16)}{(0.0952/2 + 0 + 0.305)} 10^{-1.52/0.445} 10^{-0/0.21}$$

$$H = 0.0221 \ \mu Sv/s = 7.96 \text{ mrem/hr.}$$

Laminated Primary Shield

A thin primary shield is sometimes required for treatment rooms located under an occupied area or for existing rooms that are being upgraded to accept a higher energy accelerator. In some cases the total thickness of the primary shield may be limited to 1 m or less. McGinley and Butker (1994) have reported that a laminated shield consisting of layers of lead and concrete or polyethylene can be used to produce a primary shield whose total thickness is 1.16 m. In designing such a

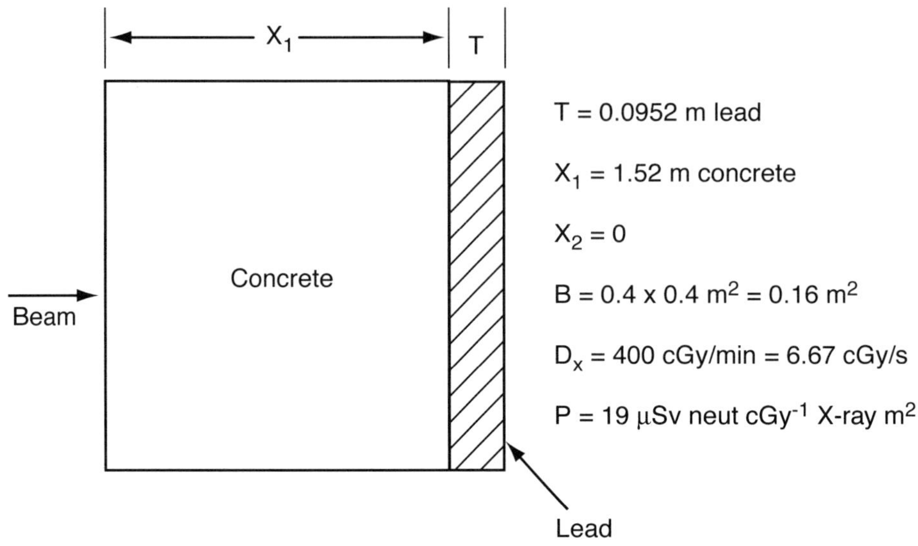

Figure 6-4. Composite shield

shield one must take into consideration the x-rays transmitted through the shield and the photoneutron and capture gamma rays produced in the shield. The following steps were used to design a thin ceiling shield for an 18 MeV accelerator:

1. The thickness of the first layer of concrete is set at 0.305 m in order to acquire sufficient structural strength.
2. The amount of lead and concrete needed to attenuate the primary beam x-ray beam to one-half the protection level is calculated using the method outlined in chapter 2.
3. The neutron level at the top of the shield is evaluated using equation 6-1.
4. If the neutron plus the photon dose equivalent is greater than the protection level, polyethylene and/or concrete is added above the lead slab.
5. The x-ray dose above the shield is re-evaluated, including the attenuation produced by any added polyethylene or concrete.
6. The x-ray level is multiplied by 2.7 to account for photons produced by neutron interactions in the shield. The value of 2.7 is equivalent to the ratio of the average value of the photon dose measured above a number of ceiling shields divided by the x-ray dose calculated using the method presented in chapter 2.

7. A second lead slab is added above the polyethylene or concrete if the photon dose determined in step 6 results in a total dose equivalent exceeding the protection level.
8. The neutron dose equivalent produced by photon interactions in the second lead layer (if used) is calculated by use of equation 6-1, and polyethylene or concrete is added if required.

The tenth value layer in polyethylene for lead photoneutrons was found to be 9.6 cm by McGinley and Butker (1994). These researchers also reported that the TVL in polyethylene for photons was 37.9 cm. Using these values and the TVL value for 18 MV x-rays, the shield design given in Table 6-1 was determined.

Table 6-1 Primary ceiling shield for 18 MeV accelerator facility*

Accelerator	*Layer number*	*Shielding material*	*Thickness (m)*
Varian 2100 C	1	concrete	0.305
	2	lead	0.203
	3	polyethylene	0.178
	4	concrete	0.305
	5	lead	0.051
	6	concrete	0.114

*The shielding materials are listed from inside the room to the floor above the accelerator. The beam size is 40 × 40 cm^2 at the isocenter. The distance from the target to the floor above is 3.64 m when the beam is aimed up.

A radiation survey of the ceiling shield indicated that the calculated and measured neutron and photon levels agreed within 5%. The following is a sample calculation for the shield given in Table 6-1.

Example Calculation

1. The first layer of concrete is made 0.305 m thick for structural strength.
2. The total number of tenth value layers needed for x-rays is now calculated based on methods explained in chapter 2 and a protection level of 1 mrem per week (half of the accepted value of 2 mrem/wk).

d = 3.64 m W = 50,000 cGy/wk at the isocenter
U = 1/4 T = 1

$$B = \frac{Pd^2}{WUT} = \frac{(1)(3.64)^2}{(50{,}000 \times 1000)(1/4)(1)} = 1.06 \times 10^{-6}$$

number of tenth value layers for photons = 1/log B = 5.97

Now we add layer 2, which is composed of lead, and have enough space left over for neutron shielding.

3. The neutron dose equivalent above layer 2 is given by:

$$H = \frac{D_X PBU}{T/2 + X_2 + 0.305} 10^{-X_1/0.455} 10^{-X_2/0.21}$$

where

$D_X = 50{,}000$ cGy/wk
$X_2 = 0$
$X_1 = 0.305$ m concrete
$X_2 = 0$ U = 1/4
B = 0.16 m^2 beam area at isocenter
T = 0.203 m lead

and

H = 0.0193 Sv/wk = 1930 mrem/wk.

This is too high, so neutron shielding must be added above layer 2.

4. Polyethylene 0.178 m thick is used above the lead. This will give the following number of TVLNs.
TVLN = 0.178 m/0.096 m = 1.85

The next layer is 0.305 m concrete and the number of TVLN is:
TVLN = 0.305 m/0.21 m = 1.45
Total TVLN = 3.30.

This gives a neutron transmission of $10^{-3.30}$ = 0.00050, and the neutron dose on top of the ceiling slab becomes
H = (1930) (0.00050) = 0.97 mrem/wk.

5. We will now check the photon dose on top of the shield.
   First evaluate the total number of tenth value layers for photons.
   layer 1 = 0.305/0.445 = 0.690
   layer 2 = 0.203/0.0556 = 3.650
   layer 3 = 0.178/0.379 = 0.470
   layer 4 = 0.305/0.445 = 0.690
   Total TVLX = 5.50

The photon dose per week is given by

$D_x = W\ U\ B/d^2 = (5.0 \times 10^7)(1/4)\ (3.16 \times 10^{-6})\ (1/3.64)^2$

$D_x = 3.0$ mrem/wk.

6. The photon dose must be corrected for the production of gamma rays in the polyethylene and concrete.
   Corrected photon dose/wk = $2.7 \times D_x = 2.7 \times 3.0 = 8.1$ mrem/wk

7. A lead layer 0.051 m thick is added to reduce the photon dose to the value shown below.
   Photon dose/wk = $(8.1)\ (10^{-0.917}) = 0.98$ mrem/wk

8. Calculation of the neutron dose equivalent/wk produced by layer 5 yields a value less than 0.01 mrem/wk. Therefore, the shield should be adequate. Since space was left over and concrete was available, layer 6 of 0.114 m thickness was added. A radiation survey of this shield resulted in values close to those calculated in this example.

A number of laminated primary barriers have been found by the author that did not provide adequate shielding. Table 6-2 summarizes the results of radiation surveys carried out at four facilities with such barriers. The x-ray MV is based on data given in the British Journal of Radiology Supplement No. 11 (1972).

Table 6-2 Radiation dose equivalent rate outside four primary barriers for an x-ray dose rate of 6.67 cGy s^{-1} at the isocenter*

X-ray beam (MV)	*Distance from target to outside of shield (m)*	*Shield material*	*Thickness (m)*	*Neutron dose equiv. rate (nSv s^{-1})*	*Photon dose equiv. rate (nSv s^{-1})*
18	3.65	concrete	0.457	116.0	55.6
		lead	0.203		
		concrete	0.254		
18	3.05	concrete	0.305	1670.0	224.0
		lead	0.203		
		concrete	0.203		
15	3.36	lead	0.025	420.0	31.1
		concrete	0.457		
		lead	0.229		
		concrete	0.076		
12	3.36	concrete	0.711	48.9	6.7
		lead	0.117		
		concrete	0.086		
		lead	0.102		

*The beam size at the isocenter was 0.4 x 0.4 m^2 for all accelerators except the 15 MeV unit which had a beam size of 0.35 x 0.35 m^2.

Patient Neutron Dose

When the metal portion of the primary barrier is placed on the inside of the treatment room, the patient will experience an increased total body radiation dose due to the production of photoneutrons when the beam strikes the shield. Measurements of the neutron dose equivalent at the patient position for two treatment rooms have been reported by McGinley (1992b). As shown in figure 6-5, each room had a metal slab on one primary wall and another wall composed of concrete. A steel slab 14 cm thick was used in one room, and lead 20 cm thick was used in the other room. Both rooms housed an 18 MeV medical accelerator with the isocenter located midway between the primary walls. A moderated activation neutron dosimeter was used for all measurements.

Neutron dose equivalent measurements were made at fixed points in the treatment room with the beam intercepting the metal-containing barrier and then the all-concrete barrier. Subtracting the measurement with the beam on the concrete wall from the value measured with the beam striking the metal-containing wall yields the dose equivalent produced by neutrons generated in the metal shielding. This procedure was carried out for points A, B, B′, C, C′, and D of figure 6-5. These points are located on a circle with a 1 m radius, centered on the isocenter of the accelerator. Maximum beam size ($0.4 \times 0.4\ m^2$) was used when the measurements were carried out. A second set of measurements was made near each wall barrier in order to simulate the situation in which total body photon treatment is carried out with the patient located near a primary wall.

It was found that the total body dose to a patient on the treatment table was increased by as much as 42% when lead was used in one primary barrier. For the same configuration, the use of steel in one primary barrier produced an increase in the neutron total body dose of 10% or less. When total body photon treatment was carried out, the neutron dose equivalent was found to be increased by a factor of 2.3 for the lead barrier and a factor of 1.2 for the steel barrier as compared with the concrete barrier.

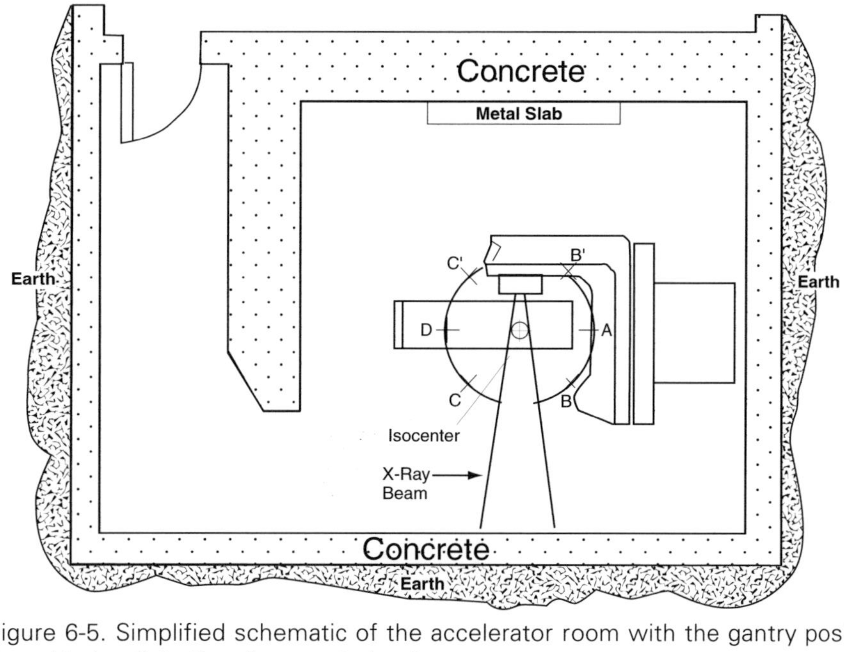

Figure 6-5. Simplified schematic of the accelerator room with the gantry positioned to irradiate the all-concrete barrier

Problems

1. Repeat example 1 with the lead placed on the inside of the treatment room.
2. Repeat example 1 with the lead replaced with a quantity of steel that has the same shielding effect for x-rays as the lead.
3. Determine the photon dose rate outside the shield of example 1. Note that the x-ray dose rate at the isocenter is 400 cGy/min. The distance from the target to the point protected is 4 m.
4. Design a tapered shield based on example 2 for situations in which the beam is angled 30° off the vertical up direction.

7

Special Topics

Radiation Skyshine

Some radiation facilities are designed with little shielding in the ceiling above the accelerator. A problem may then arise as a result of the radiation scattered by the atmosphere to points at ground level outside the treatment room. Stray radiation of this type is referred to as skyshine, and the National Council on Radiation Protection and Measurements Report No. 51 (NCRP 1977) gives methods for the calculation of skyshine for accelerator facilities.

McGinley (1993b) has compared skyshine measurements made at an 18 MeV medical accelerator facility with values calculated using the techniques presented in NCRP Report No. 51. Measurements were made of the neutron and photon levels outside a treatment room housing a Varian 2100C. The roof above the accelerator was designed for weather protection only and offered little shielding for the primary beam and scattered radiation. The distance from the treatment room floor to the roof was 4.27 m, and the primary walls were constructed of concrete 2.22 m thick. The secondary walls were fabricated of concrete 0.99 m thick. Figures 7-1 and 7-2 show vertical section views of the treatment room shielding.

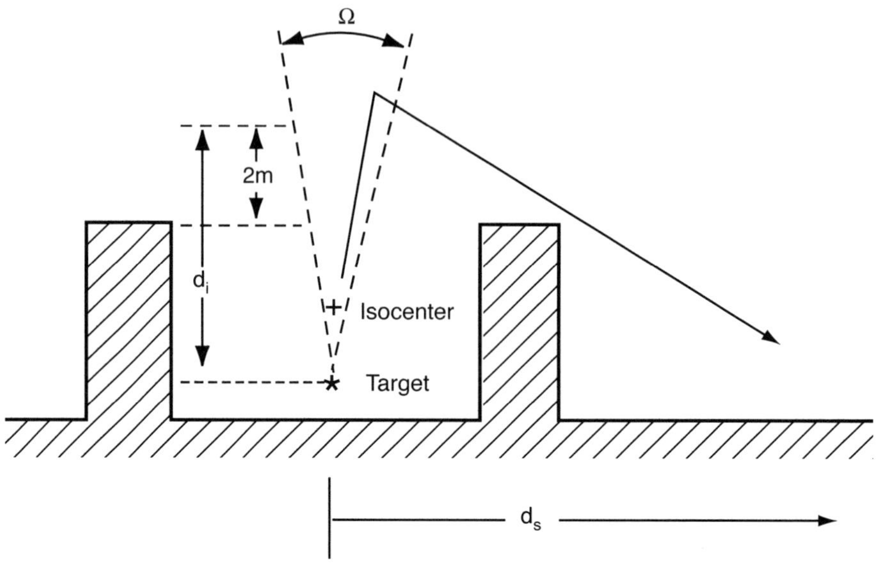

Figure 7-1. Simplified schematic showing the accelerator isocenter and target location for photon skyshine evaluation

An ionization chamber survey instrument was used to measure the photon dose with the accelerator operating at a rate of 6.67 cGy s^{-1} at a distance of 1 m from the target. In order to produce maximum skyshine, the beam was directed vertically up and the collimator was opened to maximum size (40 × 40 cm^2 at the isocenter). The x-ray dose was measured outside the accelerator room at 1 m above ground.

A neutron remmeter was used for the area survey outside the treatment room. Maximum skyshine was produced by closing the collimators and positioning the accelerator head at minimum distance from the roof, as shown in figure 7-2. The accelerator dose rate was set at 6.67 cGy s^{-1} at the isocenter.

NCRP Report No. 51 gives the following equation for calculation of the photon component of the skyshine radiation field.

$$B_{XS} = 4.02 \times 10^{-6} \frac{D(d_i d_s)^2}{(D_{io}\Omega^{1.3})} \qquad (7\text{-}1)$$

where

D = photon dose equivalent rate at ground level (nSv s^{-1})
d_s = distance (m) from isocenter to the point where the dose equivalent rate is D

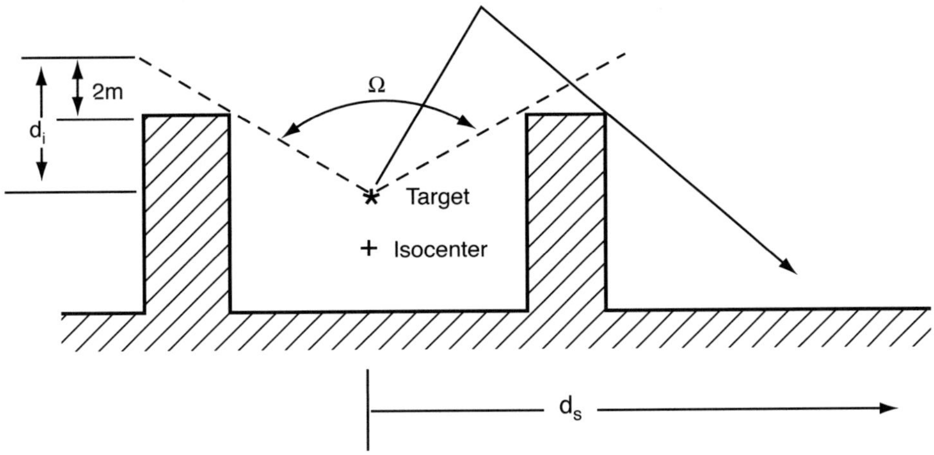

Figure 7-2. Irradiation conditions for the neutron skyshine evaluation

d_i = distance (m) from x-ray target to a point 2 m above the roof
D_{io} = x-ray dose rate at 1 m from the target (cGy s^{-1})
Ω = solid angle of radiation beam (steradians)
B_{xs} = roof shielding transmission ratio.

Equation 7-1 is based on measurements made near Cs-137 and Co-60 sources placed in a hole in the ground. Solving equation 7-1 for the skyshine dose equivalent rate gives equation 7-2.

$$D = 0.249 \times 10^6 \frac{B_{xs} D_{io} \Omega^{1.3}}{(d_i d_s)^2} \tag{7-2}$$

The following equation is given in NCRP Report No. 51 (NCRP 1977) for neutron skyshine.

$$B_{ns} = 1.19 \times 10^{-5} \frac{H d_i^2}{\Phi_o \Omega} \tag{7-3}$$

where

H = nSv s^{-1} due to neutrons at ground level
B_{ns} = roof shielding transmission ratio for neutrons
d_i = distance from target to ceiling plus 2 m
Φ_o = neutron fluence rate (cm^{-2} s^{-1}) at 1 m from the target
Ω = solid angle of shield walls.

Equation 7-3 is to be used for distances d_s less than 20 m and is based on measurements made at a research accelerator. Solving for the neutron skyshine dose equivalent rate, H, gives the following equation.

$$H = 0.84 \times 10^5 \frac{B_{ns} \Phi_o \Omega}{d_i^2} \quad (7\text{-}4)$$

Example Calculation

1. Photon Skyshine

The following parameters are used for the room shown in figure 7-1 when the photon skyshine level is calculated.

B_{xs} = 1.0 (no ceiling shield)
d_s = 10.6 m
D_{io} = 6.67 cGy s^{-1}
d_i = 5.97 m
Ω = 0.122 ster

The solid angle for a beam (see figure 7-3) with a circular cross section is $\Omega = 2\pi\,(1 - \cos\theta)$, where θ is 11.3° for a 40 x 40 cm^2 beam (which is a good assumption for the maximum collimator opening).

Introducing the values into equation 7-2 gives:

$D = 0.249 \times 10^6\,(1 \times 6.67 \times 0.122^{1.3})\,/\,(5.97 \times 10.6)^2$
$D = 26.9$ nSv s^{-1}.

2. Neutron Skyshine

The following values are used in equation 7-4.

B_{ns} = 3.36 x 10^{-10} Sv cm^{-2} (from NCRP Report No. 51 for no ceiling shielding and a neutron energy of 1.7 MeV).

Φ_o = 6.6 x 10^5 cm^{-2} s^{-1} at 1 m from the target when the x-ray dose rate is 6.67 cGy s^{-1}. This value is based on measurements made by the author for several 18 MeV accelerators.

Ω = 2.71 ster (see figure 7-2). The distance from the floor to the isocenter is 1.3 m, and the wall height is 4.97 m. The distance from the isocenter to the wall is 3.86 m. Note that the solid angle is based on the room size and not the beam size when the neutron skyshine is determined.

d_i = 4.67 m

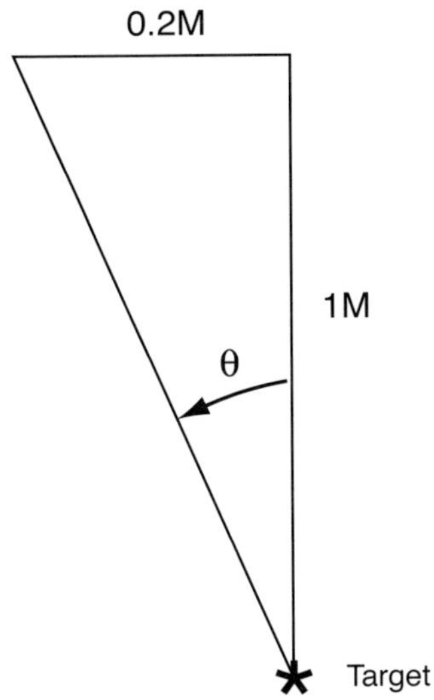

Figure 7-3. Beam geometry

From equation 7-4 we have

$H = 0.84 \times 10^5 \ (3.36 \times 10^{-10}) \ (6.6 \times 10^5) \ (2.71)/4.67^2$

$H = 2.3$ nSv s^{-1} for all points from the outer wall surface to 20 m from the isocenter.

Table 7-1 shows the measured and calculated photon skyshine dose rates as a function of distance from the isocenter (d_i). As can be seen, the measured values increase as one moves away from the wall (reaching a maximum at a distance of 13.6 m from the isocenter) and decrease as one moves past the point of maximum dose. This behavior is caused by the increase in the scattering cross section with a decreased scattering angle. A rule of thumb says that the maximum dose rate should occur at a distance from the outer wall surface that is equivalent to the wall height. Note that the calculated values continually decrease with distance from the isocenter. As shown in Table 7-1, the agreement between the calculated and measured values is poor; for distances greater than about 10 m from the isocenter, the NCRP method underestimates the photon dose rate. Table 7-2 gives the neutron skyshine levels measured with the accelerator operating at a dose rate of 6.67 cGy s^{-1} at the isocenter. At all points the measured neutron dose equivalent rate exceeded the value of 2.3 nSv s^{-1} predicted by the NCRP method.

Table 7-1 Measured and calculated x-ray skyshine for an 18 MeV accelerator with no ceiling shield*

Distance from isocenter d_s (meters)	*Measured photon rate (nSv s^{-1})*	*Calculated photon rate (nSv s^{-1})*	*Ratio measured/calculated*
7.5 (at wall)	13.9	56.2	0.25
9.4	31.2	35.4	0.88
10.6	41.7	26.9	1.5
13.6	43.7	17.4	2.5
19.2	27.8	8.3	3.3
25.4	20.8	4.9	4.2
33.0	15.3	2.9	5.3
48.3	6.9	1.3	5.3

*Dose rate at isocenter 6.67 cGy s^{-1}, beam size 40 x 40 cm^2, and beam directed vertically up.

Table 7-2 Measured neutron skyshine for an 18 MeV accelerator with no ceiling shielding*

Distance from isocenter d_s (meters)	*Measured neutron dose equivalent rate (nSv s^{-1})*
5.14	19
8.50	58
11.2	52
14.3	42
17.3	36
18.9	29
20.8	23

*Dose rate at isocenter 6.67 cGy s^{-1} with collimators closed.

The author has made neutron and photon measurements at two 18 MeV accelerators, each with a 0.91 m thick concrete ceiling slab. For each room, the radiation at ground level was found to be less than 0.4 nSv s^{-1} for both neutrons and photons. For these measurements the accelerator was operated at a dose rate of 6.67 cGy s^{-1}, and the beam was directed up.

Problems

1. Determine the neutron and photon dose equivalent rates due to skyshine for the accelerator room of problem 7 in chapter 2 at one wall height outside the east wall. Assume that there is no ceiling shielding and that the accelerator produces an 18 MV x-ray beam. The dose rate at the isocenter is 400 cGy min^{-1}, and the beam size is 40×40 cm^2.

2. What is the minimum ceiling concrete thickness needed for the accelerator room, described in the example given in this chapter, that will meet the requirement of 2 mrem for one week of operation for uncontrolled areas? Assume that the workload is 1×10^5 cGy per week and that the use factor is 1/4 for the up direction. Use the measured values for the calculation.

HVAC Openings

A rather large opening is needed in the secondary barrier for the HVAC duct to enter the treatment room. In most cases this opening is approximately 0.4×1.2 m^2 in cross section above the maze door. Table 7-3 shows typical values of the neutron and photon dose equivalent rates at the surface of the HVAC duct for several mazes of different lengths (d_2 of figure 5-1). Each room housed an 18 MeV accelerator, and the measurements were made with a dose rate of 400 cGy s^{-1} at the isocenter and the collimator open to 0.4×0.4 m^2 size.

As can be seen from Table 7-3, the radiation level adjacent to the HVAC duct is low if the maze length (d_2) is on the order of 5 m. For a short maze with d_2 less than 3 m, a shielding baffle may be needed at the HVAC penetration. Figure 7-4 shows several designs that can be used to shield the opening for the HVAC duct. The duct wrap technique, which is shown in figure 7-4, includes surrounding the duct on all sides with the shielding material, starting at the point where the duct enters the maze and ending at a point 1.2 to 1.5 m down the maze. For a high-energy accelerator, 1.0 cm of lead and 2.54 cm of polyethylene are commonly used to enclose the duct, and a low-energy accelerator needs about 0.6 cm of lead to shield the duct. A dose equivalent reduction of approximately a factor of four for neutrons and a factor of two for photons will be produced by a 1.2 m long

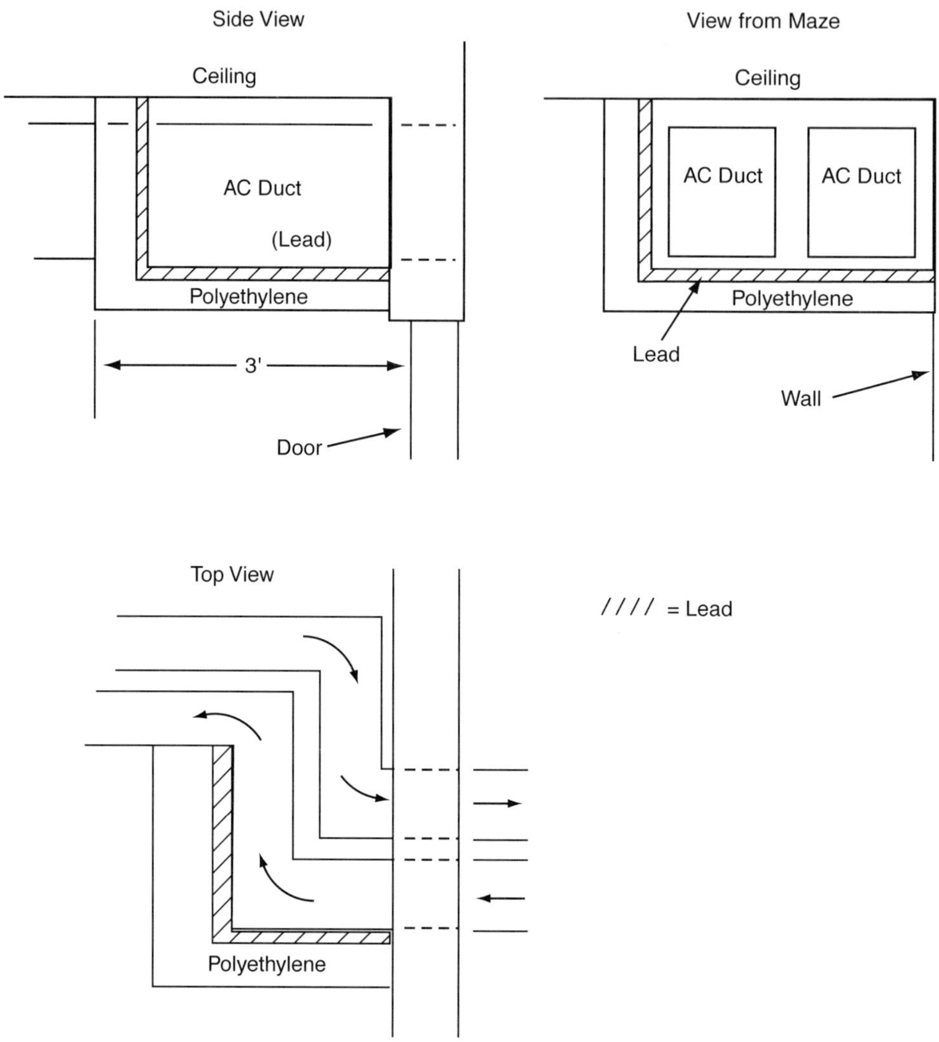

A.

Figure 7-4. HVAC duct shields. A. HVAC baffle. B. Concrete baffle. C. Duct wrap.

duct wrap shield composed of 2.54 cm of polyethylene and 1.0 cm of lead for a maze with d_2 equal to 3.6 m. As can be seen from Table 7-3, the neutron and photon dose equivalent rates change with the beam direction, and the maximum radiation level is produced by locating the accelerator head as close as possible to the maze inner opening (beam on wall A).

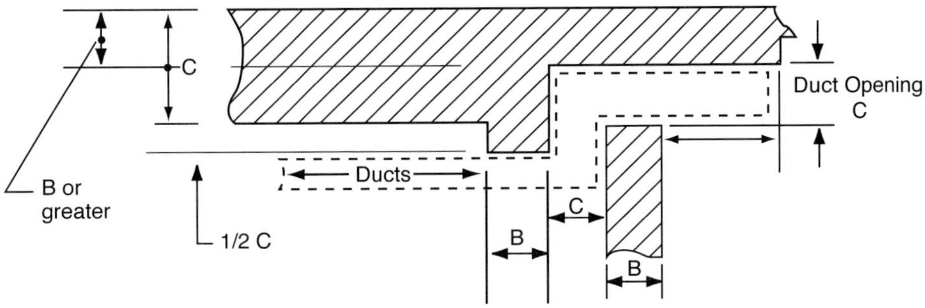
C
B or
greater
1/2 C
Ducts
B
C
B
Duct Opening
C

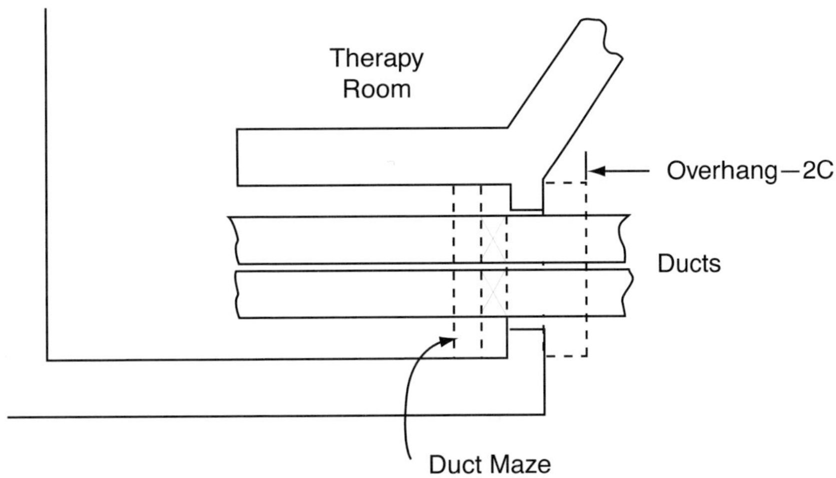
Therapy
Room
Overhang—2C
Ducts
Duct Maze

B.

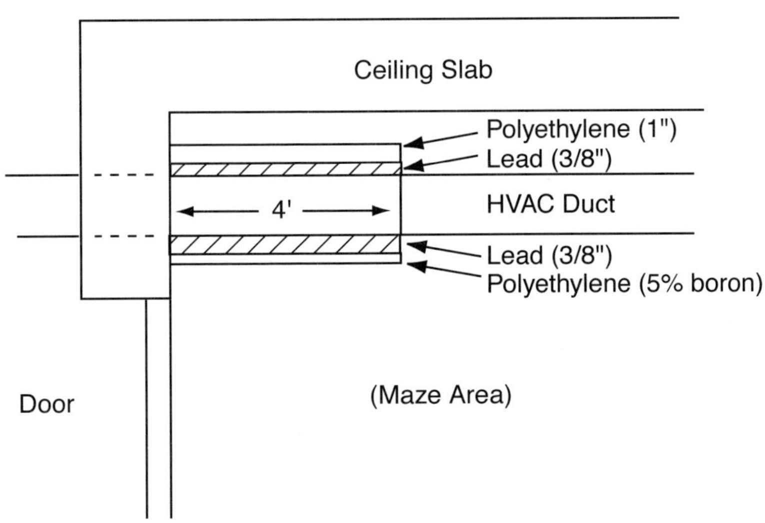
Ceiling Slab
Polyethylene (1")
Lead (3/8")
4'
HVAC Duct
Lead (3/8")
Polyethylene (5% boron)
Door
(Maze Area)

C.

Table 7-3 Neutron and photon dose equivalent levels adjacent to the HVAC duct*

Room	*Beam direction*†	*Neutron dose equivalent (nSv s^{-1})*	*Photon dose equivalent (nSv s^{-1})*	*d_1 (m)*	*d_2 (m)*
1	down	1.22	2.77	5.2	5.2
	on wall C	2.22	1.67		
	on wall A	1.66	3.33		
	up	1.39	2.60		
2	down	9.16	15.3	5.2	2.2
	on wall C	13.9	9.72		
	on wall A	31.7	22.2		
	up	8.72	13.7		

*The dose rate at the isocenter is 6.67 cGy s^{-1} and the field is 0.4 × 0.4 m^2. None of the HVAC ducts are shielded.
†See figure 3-1 for beam directions.

Figure 7-4 also shows a shadow shield and a concrete wall baffle for the HVAC penetration. The shadow shield requires about the same thickness of shielding material as the duct wrap method. The duct is mounted near the ceiling slab and only the bottom and two sides are shielded. In place of using a shadow shield, a concrete wall baffle can be placed above the maze door to reduce the radiation level at the HVAC opening. Note that in figure 7-4 the dimension (C), which is the height of the duct, is also related to several of the baffle dimensions.

Ozone Production

Ozone (O_3) is produced by radiation interactions with oxygen (O_2) in the air of the treatment room. If a medical linear accelerator is operated in the electron mode, more ozone is produced than when the photon mode is used. Ozone is considered an injurious and potentially lethal gas at a level of a few parts per million (ppm), and a maximum permissible concentration (MPC) of 0.1 ppm has been recommended (NCRP 1977). The odor produced by a concentration of 0.1 ppm is detectable by most individuals. The concentration, C, of ozone in ppm after the accelerator has been operated for a length of time, t, is given by

$$H = \frac{C_o G E S_{col} \, Id}{NV(Q/V)} \times (1 - e^{-(Q/V)t}) \times 10^9 \qquad (7\text{-}5)$$

where

C_o = fraction by weight of O_2 in air (0.232)

G = ozone production by electron irradiation of air (approximately 6 molecules per 100 electron volts)

E = the number of electronic charges per milliamp per second of electron beam current (6.28×10^{15} mA^{-1} s^{-1})

S_{col} = collision stopping power of the electron (about 2.7 KeV cm^{-1} from 2 to 25 MeV)

I = average external electron beam current (mA)

d = distance of travel of the electrons in air (cm)

N = Avogadro's number (6.02×10^{23} molecules per 22.4 liters air)

V = room volume in liters

Q = room ventilation rate (liters s^{-1})

Q/V = number of room air changes per second

t = irradiation time(s).

In deriving equation 7-5 it has been assumed that there is no dissociation of the ozone during the irradiation. If we consider a 6 MeV electron beam with an average external beam current of 2 microampere, 100 cm beam travel, a room volume of 100,000 liters, and a ventilation rate of greater than six room changes per hour, we find that the MPC level of ozone will not be reached for an infinitely long irradiation. When total skin electron therapy is performed with a low-energy electron beam, travel distances of approximately three meters and high beam currents are used, which can produce greater levels of ozone than the example given above. However, for normal clinical use of electron beams, a room ventilation rate of about three room changes per hour is more than adequate for health protection. The ozone level produced by photon beams is in general less than that due to electron beams.

Example Calculation

Determine the time required to reach the MPC for ozone for a 1×10^5 liter room volume and an electron beam current of 20 μA. The beam path length in air is 100 cm, and the ventilation rate is 2.0 room changes per hour.

Expressing Q/V in room changes per s gives

$$Q/V = 2.0/3600 = 5.56 \times 10^{-4}\ s^{-1}.$$

From equation 7-5 we have

$$H = \frac{C_O GES_{col} Id}{NV(Q/V)} \times (1\text{-}e^{-(Q/V)t})(10^9)$$

$$0.1 = \frac{(0.232)(6/100)(6.28\times10^{15})(2.7)(2\times10^{-2})(100)(1\text{-}e^{-2t})(10^9)}{(6.02\times10^{23}/22.4)(1\times10^5)(5.56\times10^{-4})}$$

and solving for t gives

$$t = 0.19 \text{ hours} = 11.4 \text{ minutes}.$$

Problem

Determine the ozone concentration for the room described above 10 minutes after the end of a 11.4 minute irradiation.

Air Activation

Air is made radioactive by medical linear accelerators operating above 10 MeV primarily by the photoneutron reactions shown below.

$^{14}N(\gamma,n)^{13}N$	half-life = 600 s	Threshold = 10.5 MeV
$^{16}O(\gamma,n)^{15}O$	half-life = 122 s	Threshold = 15.7 MeV

Each reaction produces a positron emitter with a relatively short half-life. The patient and radiotherapy technologist are exposed to positrons and annihilation photons with an energy of 0.511 MeV. Table 7-4 presents the maximum permissible concentration in air (MPC_a) based on a 40-hour work week and the typical volume of a treatment room. As can be seen from Table 7-4, the limiting condition for air activation is due to skin irradiation by positrons from oxygen and nitrogen.

Table 7-4 MPC$_a$ values and dose limits (D$_l$) for air activation products

Isotope	*Organ*	*MCA$_a$ (Bq m^{-3})*	*D$_l$ (nSv s^{-1})*	*Radiation type*
^{13}N	skin	1.48 x 10^6	41.7	positrons
^{13}N	whole body	0.85 x 10^7	6.95	annihilation
^{15}O	skin	0.74 x 10^6	41.7	positrons
^{15}O	whole body	0.85 x 10^7	6.95	annihilation

The activity of ^{13}N or ^{15}O per unit volume of air (C) produced in the treatment room by a 20 × 20 cm^2 beam is given by equation 7-6 (McGinley et al. 1984).

$$C = \frac{(D/16.7)\,(P)\,(1-e^{-(\lambda + Q/V)T_r})\,(e^{-(\lambda + Q/V)T_s})}{V(\lambda + Q/V)/\lambda} \qquad (7\text{-}6)$$

where

C = concentration (Bq m^{-3})

D = dose rate at maximum build-up depth (mGy s^{-1})

P = production rate of ^{13}N or ^{15}O at a dose rate of 16.7 mGy s^{-1} (Bq kg^{-1} of oxygen or nitrogen)

Q = room ventilation rate (m^3 s^{-1})

V = volume of room (m^3)

λ = decay constant for ^{13}N or ^{15}O (s^{-1})

T_r = irradiation time (s)

T_s = time after end of irradiation (s).

Values of the production rate (P) have been reported by McGinley et al. (1984) for betatron-produced x-ray beams. If one uses these values of P for a linear accelerator, a slight overestimation of the air concentration of ^{13}N and ^{15}O will result. Table 7-4 shows values of P for selected x-ray megavoltages (McGinley et al. 1984).

Table 7-5 Activity production rates (P) for various x-ray beams and a 0.2 x 0.2 m² field*

Megavoltage (MV)	*Isotope*	*P (Bq kg⁻¹ N₂)*	*Isotope*	*P (Bq kg⁻¹ O₂)*
15	^{13}N	1.05	^{15}O	0.00
18		2.3		0.32
20		3.0		1.0
25		6.5		6.2
33		8.1		14.0
45		10.0		15.2

*The dose rate at the isocenter is 16.7 mGy s^{-1}.

The total dose equivalent to the skin of a technologist in a year's time was calculated by McGinley et al.(1984) for the treatment of 40 patients per day, five days per week, and 4 Gy daily dose per patient. A daily treatment time of 120 s and 600 s stay time per patient was assumed for the evaluation. It was found that the skin dose equivalent was well below the maximum permissible dose equivalent of 0.5 Sv used at the time of the study and that air activation represents a minimal hazard to the technologist.

Atrium

In order to create a more pleasant atmosphere in the treatment room, a few facilities have used an atrium or skylight located in the secondary portion of the ceiling. Figure 7-5 shows a room with an atrium in the shape of a triangle with sides 5.94 m, 4.00 m, and 4.40 m in length. The accelerator was operated in the 18 MV x-ray mode with the collimator fully open (0.4×0.4 m^2) and a dose rate of 5.0 cG s^{-1} at the isocenter. The results of a radiation survey conducted with the beam directed vertically up are shown in Table 7-6. The dose equivalent rate at the outside of the atrium was on the order of 139 nSv s^{-1} for neutrons and 38 nSv s^{-1} for photons. The dose equivalent rate as one moves away from the building at ground level increases up to a distance of 16.5 m from the isocenter and then drops off with increasing distance.

The radiation level inside the building was found to increase as one moves from the first to third floor. The total dose equivalent on the third floor exceeds the limit of 0.02 mSv per week for uncontrolled

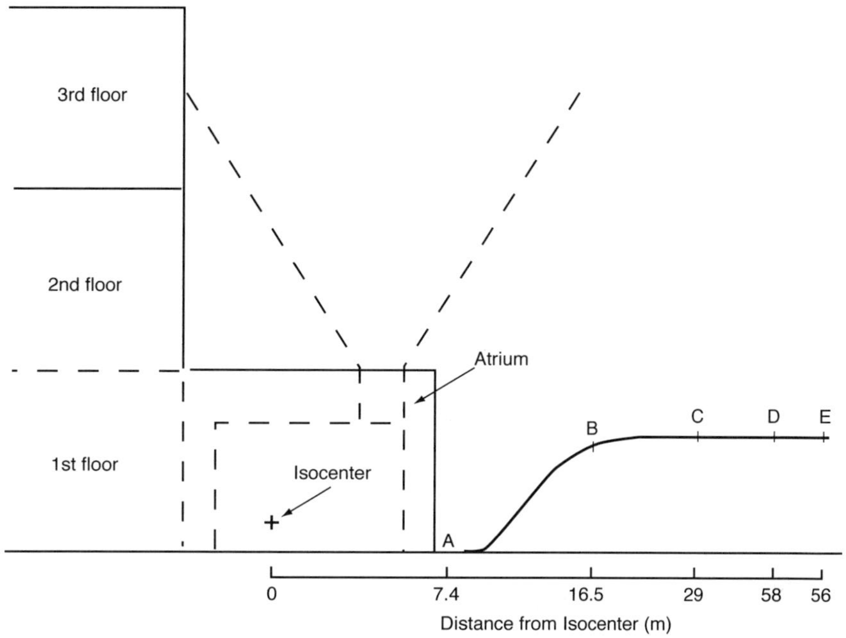

Figure 7-5. Treatment room with an atrium

areas if one assumes a workload greater than 2.8×10^4 cGy in seven days and an occupancy factor for the third floor of one.

An additional problem that is created by the use of an atrium is the high level of light in the treatment room, which may make it impossible to see the light beam representing the radiation field on the patient's skin. As a result of this problem, it may be necessary to have blinds on the atrium that automatically shut when the radiation field light is illuminated.

Alternate Shielding Materials

A number of materials other than concrete, steel, and lead can be used for radiation shielding purposes. For example, the room without a ceiling shielding that was described in the skyshine section of this chapter was modified by adding a 10 cm layer of asphalt to the roof. This material is rich in hydrogen, so it is a good fast neutron shield and the slow neutron flux will be reduced by hydrogen capture reactions. However, the photon dose level will be only slightly attenuated by the asphalt. A reduction of the neutron dose equivalent by a factor

Table 7-6 Photon and neutron dose equivalent rates in the vicinity of an 18 MeV accelerator room

Location (see figure 7-5)	*Distance from isocenter (m)*	*Neutron rate ($nSv\ s^{-1}$)*	*Photon rate ($nSv\ s^{-1}$)*
A	7.4	0.39	0 .28
B	16.5	0.45	0.56
C	29.0	0.36	< 0.15
D	50.0	0.14	< 0.15
E	56.0	0.11	< 0.15
2nd floor	—	1.47	1.08
3rd floor	—	2.78	1.08

of approximately ten was observed with the asphalt roof coat in place. It would be possible to add a strong slow neutron absorber such as boron to the asphalt and enhance the slow neutron shielding properties of the material.

Water is a hydrogenous material in which a boron compound such as borax or boric acid can be dissolved. The author and co-worker Jeffrey Long have fabricated a low-cost "water" door for a treatment room by filling a stainless steel door case with borated water (U.S. Patent No. 4833335). To eliminate the possibility of water leakage and evaporation, a polyester resin that forms a gel with the water can be added. The door was placed at the inner maze entrance to prevent neutrons from entering the maze, thereby reducing the dose equivalent due to capture gammas and neutrons at the outer maze entrance. Measurements were made outside the water door, and values of 7.5 cm and 21.5 cm of water were found for the TVL for neutrons and photons, respectively. The accelerator was operated in the 20 MV x-ray mode, and the isocenter was visible from the door opening. With a moderate length maze an additional shielded door is not needed at the outer maze entrance. The total cost of the water door was approximately $2000 as compared with a typical lead and polyethylene door, which has a cost of $30,000 to $50,000.

8

Simulator, HDR, and Brachytherapy Rooms

Simulators

A simulator is an x-ray unit used to establish a treatment procedure before radiation therapy is begun. An isocentric tube mount is used so the movement of the beam will be similar to the treatment unit, and both radiographic and fluoroscopic modes of operation are possible. Recently simulators have become available that have computed tomography (CT) capabilities. Figure 8-1 shows a conventional simulator room that is used for fluoroscopy and radiography work. Most exposures are made in the fluoroscopy mode, and only a relatively small amount of radiographic work is carried out. The simulator is typically operated so that the image receptor and x-ray diaphragm move together in such a manner that the x-ray beam is collimated to conform to the image intensifier. This means that the primary beam is reduced in intensity before it intercepts a barrier due to the fact that it must pass through the image intensifier.

The techniques used for simulator shielding design are similar to those for medical accelerators with certain exceptions, noted below. Shielding is normally provided to a height of seven feet above the floor and in the ceiling if the space above is occupied. Lead-backed gypsum board is used in the walls, and the room door is made of wood with

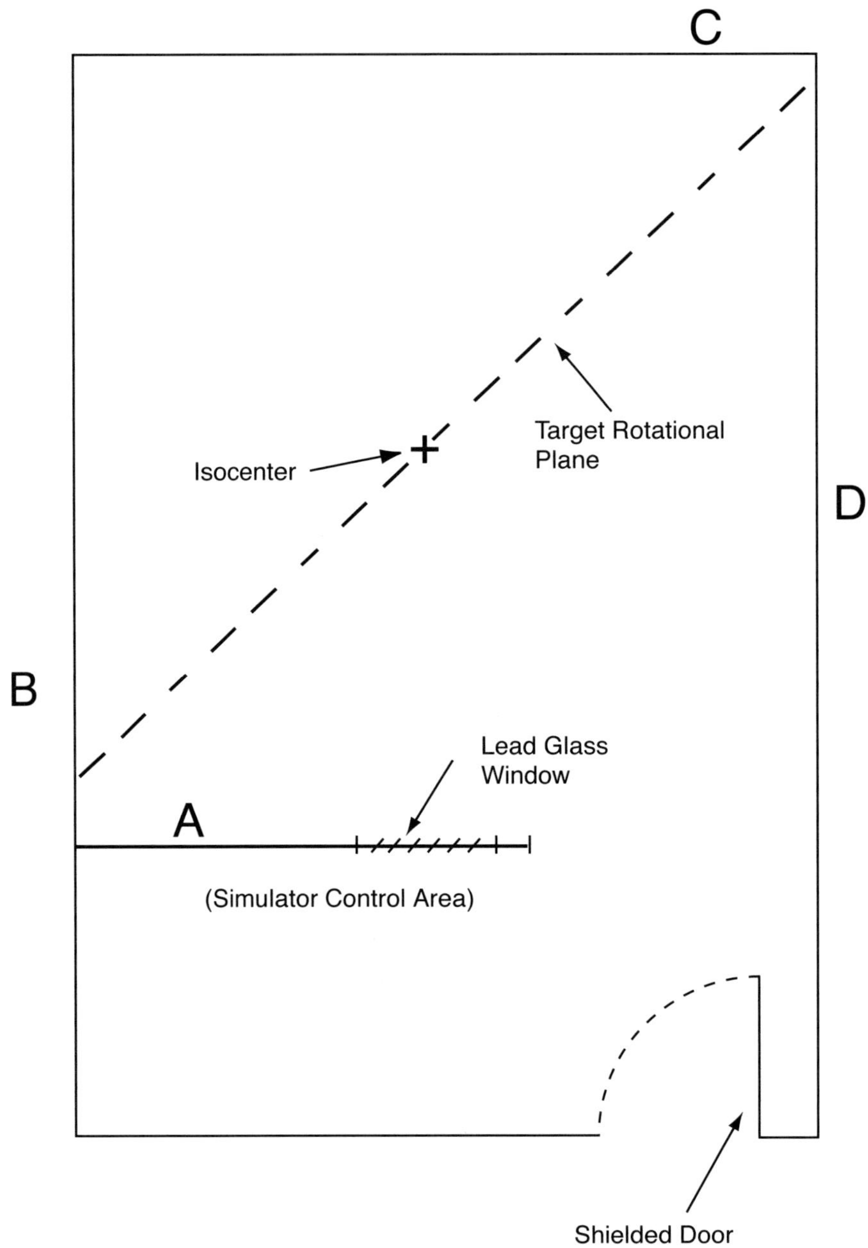

Figure 8-1. Conventional radiotherapy simulator floor plan

a lead core. A viewing window made of leaded glass is provided so the operator can see the patient during the simulation process. The workload (W) is expressed in terms of milliamperes multiplied by the exposure time in minutes (mA min), and values of 160, 300, and 3200 mA min per week are typical for radiography, fluoroscopy, and CT, respectively. Protection levels (P), use factors (U), and occupancy factors (T) for controlled and uncontrolled areas given in chapter 2 can be used for simulators.

Shielding calculations are conducted as shown below, using the methods given in NCRP Report No. 49 (NCRP 1976). For a primary barrier the exposure per mA minute (K_{ux}) in seven consecutive days of operation is computed by use of equation 8-1.

$$K_{ux} = \frac{Pd^2}{WUT} \tag{8-1}$$

where

P = protection level (R wk^{-1})
d = distance from the x-ray target to the area being protected (m)
W = workload in mA min wk^{-1}
U = use factor (1/4 for each wall, floor, and ceiling)
T = occupancy factor.

The value of K_{ux} is used with figure 8-2 to determine the thickness of lead required for the primary barrier. Figure 8-2 is based on 125 kV x-rays, which is a typical operating voltage for a radiotherapy simulator. Note that the transmission curve cannot be described by a single half value layer, and the thickness of lead needed must be determined graphically. The primary barrier will receive only scattered radiation 75% of the time. The scattered radiation can be ignored, since it will be a factor of 1000 less than the primary radiation. The width of the primary barrier is made 30 cm larger than the maximum beam size on all sides in order to reduce leakage caused by photons scattered from the main beam.

Radiation that reaches a secondary barrier is made up of patient scatter and head leakage. Shielding for each component is based on equations 8-2 and 8-5. The barrier transmission factor (B) required for head leakage is given by equation 8-2.

$$B = \frac{P(d_{sec})^2\ 600\ I}{WT} \tag{8-2}$$

where

P = protection level for area protected (R wk^{-1})

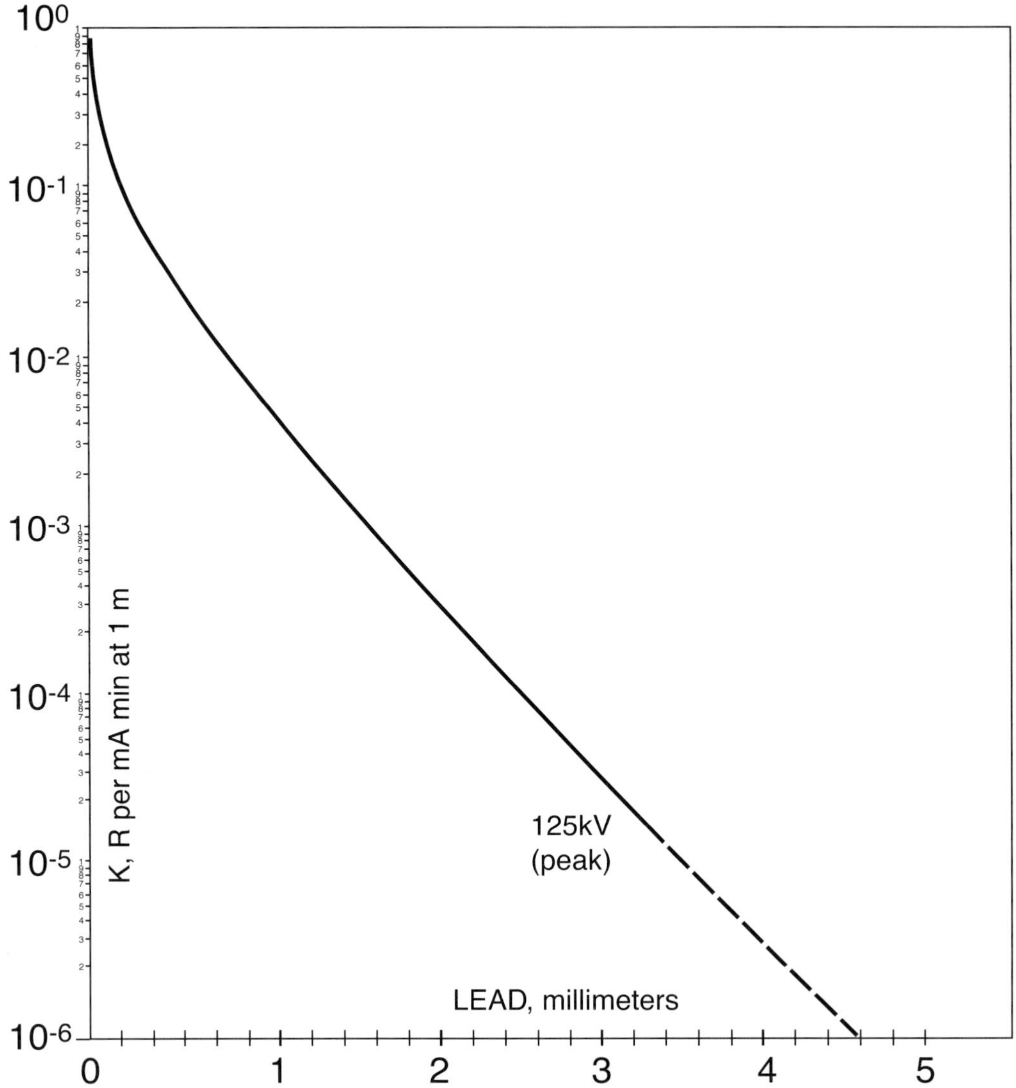

Figure 8-2. Transmission factor (K_{ux}) as a function of lead thickness for 125 kV x-ray beam. From NCRP (1976).

d_{sec} = distance in meters from radiation source to point protected

I = maximum tube current (4mA)

W = workload (mA min wk^{-1})

T = occupancy factor.

In equation 8-2 it has been assumed that the tube head leakage at one meter is 0.1 R min^{-1}. The value of B is used to compute the number of half value layers (N) required for the shield as given by equation 8-3.

$$N = 3.32 \log_{10}(1/B) \tag{8-3}$$

The shield thickness for leakage (S_L) is then calculated using equation 8-4.

$$S_L = N\ (HVL) \tag{8-4}$$

where

HVL = 0.28 mm lead for 125 kV x-ray.

Next, the barrier transmission factor (K_{ux}) for patient scatter is determined by use of equation 8-5.

$$K_{ux} = \frac{P}{aWT}(d_{sca})^2(d_{sec})^2\frac{400}{F} \tag{8-5}$$

All of the terms in equation 8-5 have the same meaning as those of equation 2-2 except the workload (W), which is in terms of mA min wk^{-1}. Values of the scattering coefficient (a) as a function of the scattering angle from the central rays for 125 kV x-ray are presented in Table 8-1. The required thickness of lead is then read from figure 8-2. If the barrier thickness based on leakage and scatter differs by a tenth value layer, the thicker is used. If the thickness differs by less than one tenth value layer, one HVL (0.28 mm lead) is added to the thicker.

Table 8-1 Patient scattering coefficients (a) for 125 kV x-ray from NCRP Report No. 49*

Angle (deg)	*30*	*45*	*60*	*90*	*120*	*135*
a	0.0018	0.0015	0.0015	0.0015	0.0023	0.0025

*From NCRP 1976.

Example Calculations

1. Evaluate the thickness of lead needed in primary wall (A) of figure 8-1. The distance from the target to the wall is 3.5 m, and the area

outside the wall is a controlled space. A workload of 400 mA min per week is used for the simulator.

Using equation 8-1 we have:

$$K_{ux} = \frac{Pd^2}{WUT}$$

$$K_{ux} = \frac{(0.01)(3.5)^2}{(400)(1/4)(1)} = 0.00122 \text{ R per mA min.}$$

Based on figure 8-2, the lead thickness needed is 1.6 mm.

2. Determine the lead shielding needed for the secondary wall (B) of figure 8-1 if the distance from the patient to the target is one meter and the distance from the isocenter to the point protected is 4.5 m. The field size at the patient is 0.3×0.3 m^2, and the area outside the wall is uncontrolled with an occupancy factor of 1/4.

   The barrier thickness for leakage radiation is based on equation 8-2.

$$B = \frac{P(d_{sec})^2\, 600(I)}{WT} = \frac{0.002(4.5)^2\, 600(4)}{400(1/4)} = 0.97$$

The number of HVL of lead needed is given below.

$$N = 3.32 \log_{10}(1/0.97) = 0.044$$

The lead thickness for head leakage is

$$S_L = N\ (HVL) = 0.044\ (0.28) = 0.012 \text{ mm of lead.}$$

Now the shielding requirement for patient scatter will be evaluated.

$$K_{ux} = \frac{P}{aWT}\,(d_{sca})^2(d_{sec})^2\,\frac{400}{F}$$

$$K_{ux} = \frac{0.002}{(0.0015)(400)(1/4)}\,(1)^2(4.5)^2\,\frac{400}{900} = 0.12 \text{ R per mA min}$$

Reading figure 8-2 for a K_{ux} value of 0.12 R per mA min yields a lead thickness of 0.1 mm. Lead shielding of 1/16″ would be used because this is the thickness available commercially for architectural use.

Problem

1. Determine the lead equivalency of the glass needed for the view window shown in figure 8-1. The distance from the isocenter to the window is 2.9 m.

HDR Rooms

High-dose-rate (HDR) afterloading units are currently used for most brachytherapy procedures. These devices allow the placement of a radioactive source in the patient after catheters have been put in place. ^{192}Ir is the most commonly used radioactive material, and a typical source has a strength of 10 Ci or less. The source is welded to a flexible cable that can be driven into the catheter by the HDR unit to selected positions.

A fully shielded room is needed to house the unit; an existing cobalt room or accelerator room can be used. Figure 8-3 depicts a treatment room dedicated to HDR treatment only. Entry into the room may be through a direct shielded door or by a short maze. Typical room shielding consists of 0.35 to 0.61 m of concrete or 4 to 5 cm of lead. The shielding requirements for the room are based on equation 8-6, where B is the barrier transmission factor.

$$B = Pd^2 / WT \tag{8-6}$$

where

P = radiation protection level for area protected
d = distance from the source to the point protected (m)
W = workload (cGy wk^{-1}, cGy yr^{-1}, or cGy in any one hour of operation at 1 m from the source)
T = occupancy factor.

The workload (W) is evaluated based on the number of patients to be treated per week, per year, or in one hour and the dose that will be delivered to each patient. For example, if 25 patient treatments are to be given per week and if each patient will receive 10 Gy at a distance of 1 cm from the source, the total treatment time (t) per week can be evaluated from the dose rate in tissue at 1 cm from the source.

$$t = \frac{(10)\,(\text{number of patients per week})}{(\text{dose rate at 1 cm})} \tag{8-7}$$

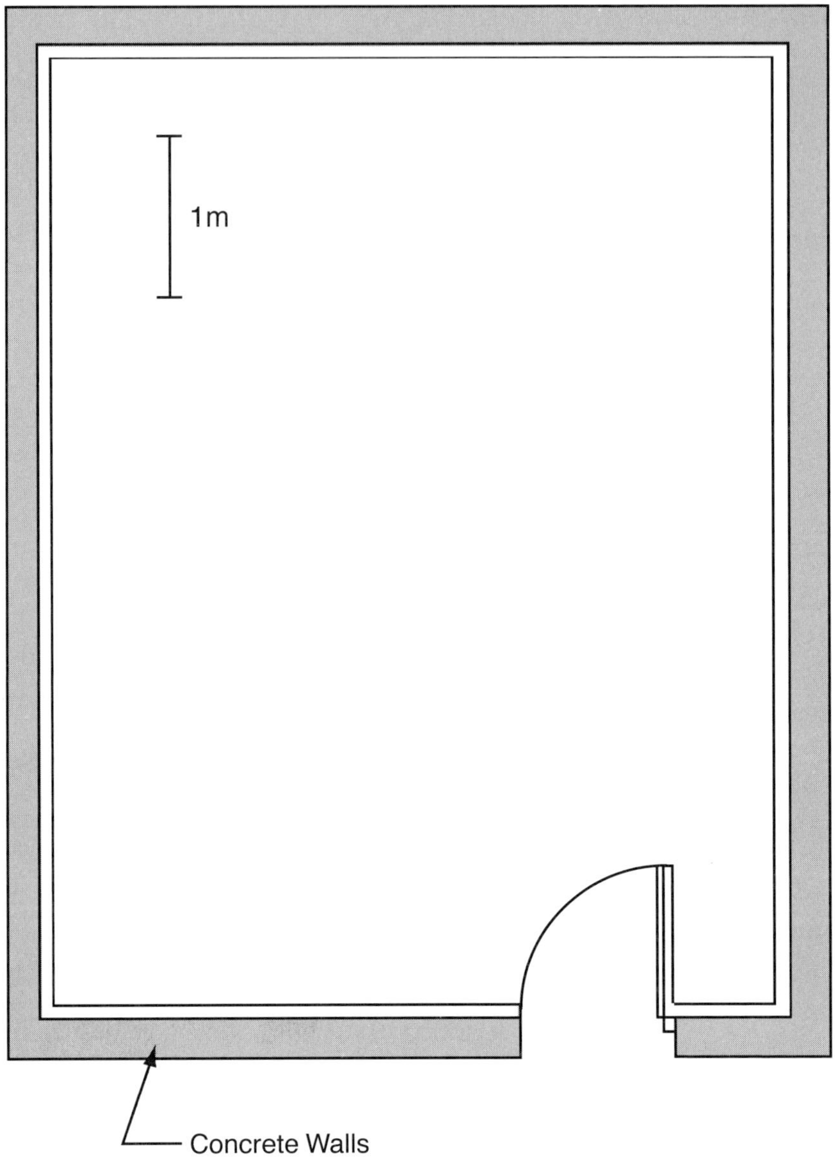

Figure 8-3. Floor plan of HDR room

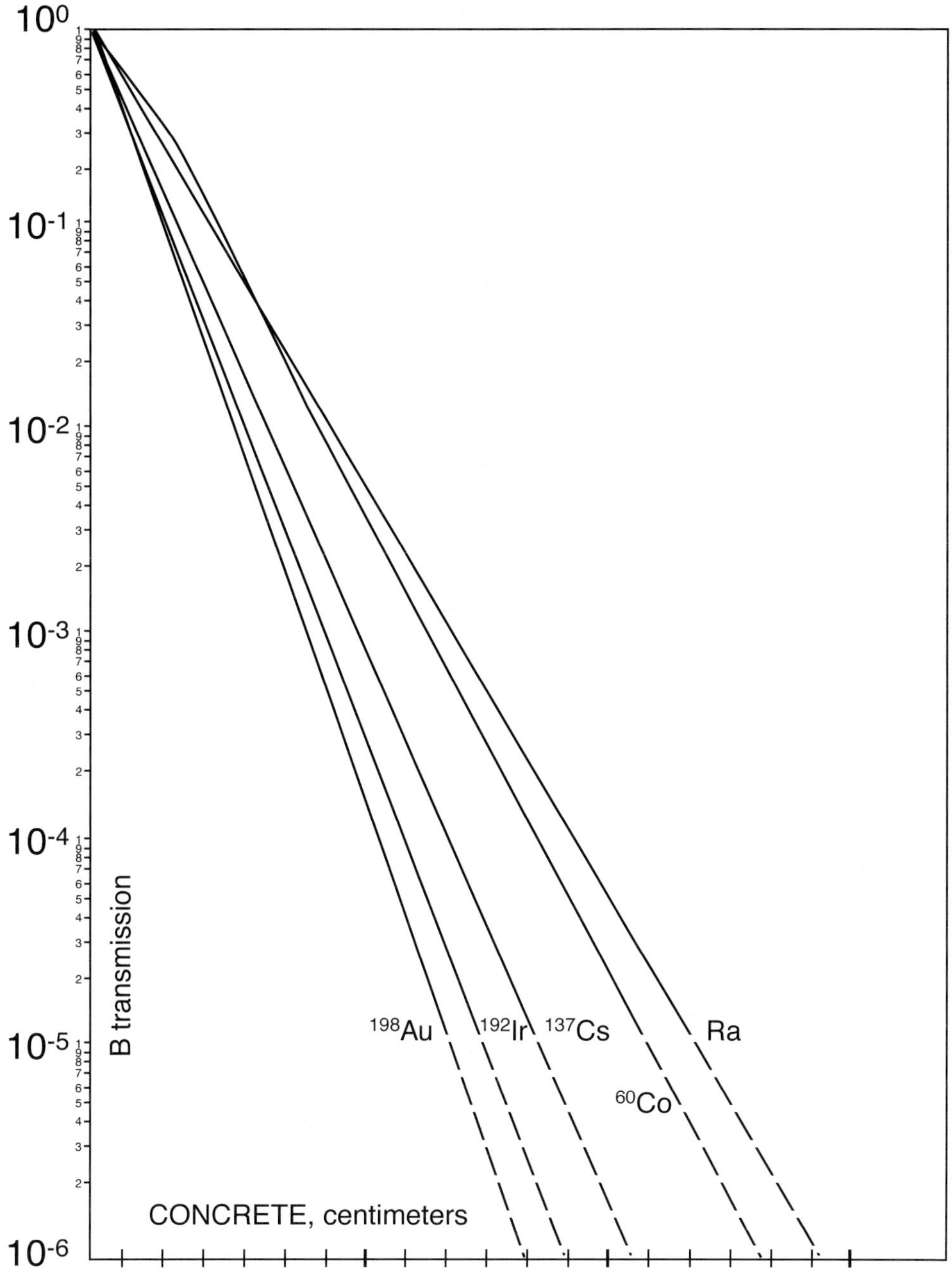

Figure 8-4. Barrier transmission factor (B) as a function of concrete thickness for various radioisotopes. From NCRP Report No. 49 (NCRP 1976) with permission.

A dose rate at 1 cm of 1 Gy per minute is typical of a 10 Ci ^{192}Ir source, so the total treatment time (t) will be 250 minutes per week. Now the workload in one week can be evaluated by equation 8-8. Based on our example the workload is 19.2 cGy per week at 1 m.

$$W = \gamma f A t \tag{8-8}$$

where

γ = gamma factor for ^{192}Ir = 0.48 R/Ci/hr at 1 m
f = f factor for ^{192}Ir = 0.96 cGy/R
A = activity of source (Ci).

If T is one and d has a value of 1.61 m, the barrier transmission factor (B) obtained by use of equation 8-6 has a value of 2.7×10^{-4} for an uncontrolled area. The thickness of concrete shielding needed is read from figure 8-4, yielding a value of 0.54 m of concrete. Leakage radiation with the source in the off position is less than 0.1 mR/hr and can be ignored when the shielding needs are evaluated.

Problem

1. Determine the thickness of lead needed in the HDR room door shown in figure 8-3.

Brachytherapy Rooms

The radiation level outside hospital rooms housing brachytherapy patients often exceeds the limits allowed by the Nuclear Regulatory Commission regulations. In particular, the exposure to the patient in the adjoining room may present a radiological health problem. Possible solutions include the use of portable shields, vacating the rooms adjacent to the brachytherapy treatment room, and shielding the walls and possibly the ceiling and floor of the room. For new construction the last solution is the best, and for an existing building the same solution can be used provided the structural strength of the floor is not exceeded. Portable shields are inconvenient to use and do not reduce the radiation intensity in all directions. Vacating rooms adjacent to brachytherapy treatment rooms is costly in terms of lost revenue as well as inconvenient. The technique for designing permanent shielding for a brachytherapy room is described below.

Figure 8-5 depicts the room to be shielded and the normal location of the radioactive sources. The position of the bed cannot be changed due to the location of the utility outlets on the room wall. A maximum patient loading of 100 mg Ra equivalent of ^{137}Cs will be used for the calculation. The dose limit to the patient in the adjoining room is assumed to be 1.0 mGy during any given admission, and the average stay time for the patient is seven days. The dose rate in uncontrolled areas such as corridors and stairways is to be restricted to 0.02 mGy per hour. For an adjacent room the dose limit applies to the patient, and for the floor above the brachytherapy room the dose is determined at floor level. The dose is limited at seven feet above the floor level for the room below, and for uncontrolled areas the dose rate is to be 0.02 mGy per hour at the outer wall surface of the brachytherapy room. The protection limits discussed here may vary depending on local and national regulations.

The barrier transmission factor (B) is calculated with equation 8-9.

$$B = Pd^2/(0.80f\gamma A) \tag{8-9}$$

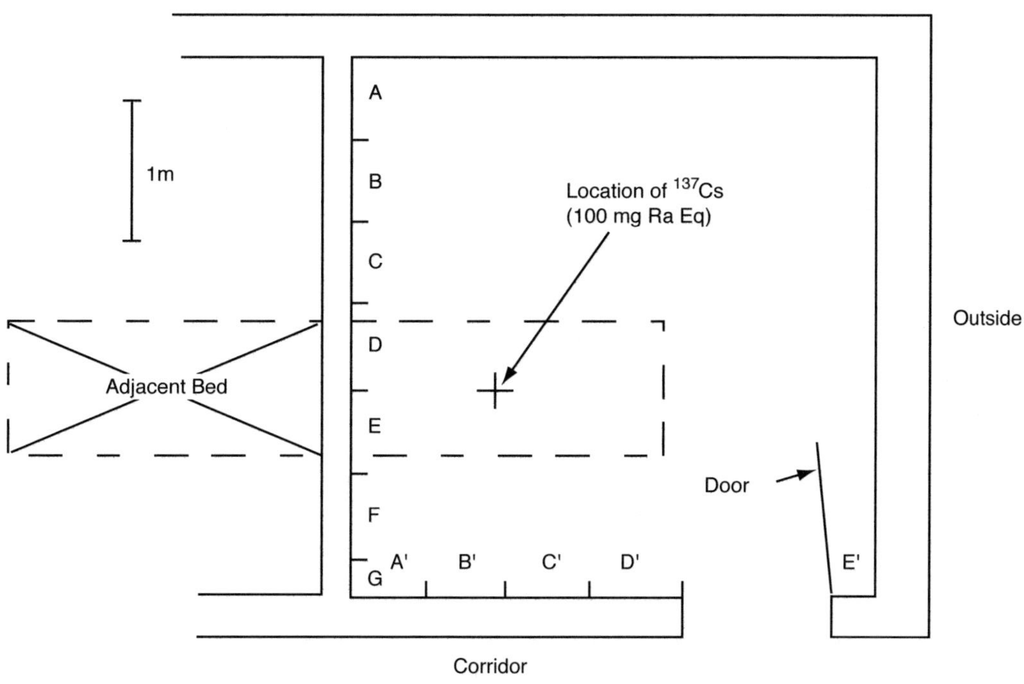

Figure 8-5. Brachytherapy room floor plan showing wall shield segments

where:

P = protection level (0.60 mcGy per hour for other nearby patients and 2 mcGy per hr for uncontrolled areas such as corridors and stairs)

d = distance to adjacent patient or distance to outer room wall (m)

0.80 = transmission through patient for ^{137}Cs radiation

f = f factor for ^{137}Cs = 0.96 cGy/R

γ = gamma factor for radium 0.825 mcGy m^2/mg hr

A = mg Ra equivalent of Cs in patient.

The thickness (S) of concrete or lead shielding is read from figure 8-4 or 8-6 (NCRP 1976). Oblique incidence of the radiation on the barrier allows reduction in the thickness of shielding required as shown by figure 8-6. A tapered barrier may be employed to reduce cost and weight. The thickness (T) of the shield is given by

$$T = S\,(\cos\theta) \tag{8-10}$$

where

S = thickness based on value of B

θ = angle of obliquity.

Example Calculation

Calculate the thickness of lead needed for wall segments D and B of figure 8-5 if the patient loading is 100 mg Ra equivalent of ^{137}Cs. Each of the wall segments is two feet wide.

1. Segment D: The barrier transmission factor (B) required for the patient in the adjoining room is given by

$$B = Pd^2/(0.80f\gamma A) = (0.60)(2.44^2)/(0.80)(0.96)(0.825)(100)$$

$$B = 0.0564.$$

From figure 8-6 we obtain a lead thickness of 2.7 cm. Since the angle θ is about 0°, the slant thickness (S) and physical thickness (T) of the barrier are approximately the same. Note that the distance (d) used for the evaluation is the distance between the bed centers. Repeating the calculation for the barrier transmission needed to protect visitors

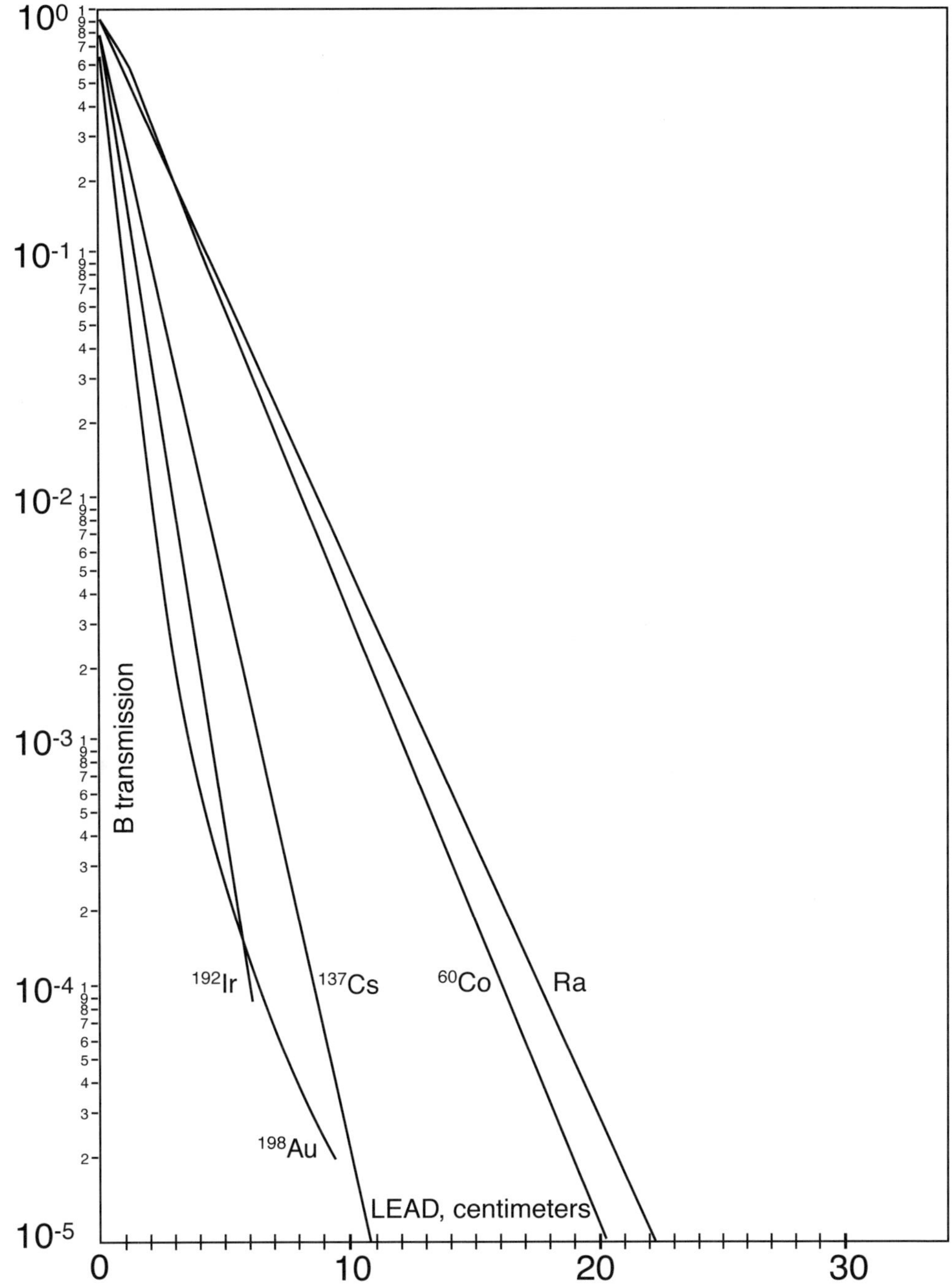

Figure 8-6. Barrier transmission factor (B) as a function of lead thickness of ^{137}Cs. From NCRP Report No. 49 (NCRP 1976).

in the adjoining room using a value of 2.0 mcGy per hr and the distance to the wall surface leads to a lead thickness of 3.0 cm, so the wall segment will be made 3.0 cm thick.

2. Segment B: The minimum value of the distance (d) from the source-to-wall segment B will be used to evaluate the required transmission (B), and the angle θ is also based on the minimum value of d in order to arrive at a conservative value of the shield thickness. From the room diagram it is found that the minimum value of d is 1.98 m and the minimum value of the angle θ is 46.2°. Solving for the transmission factor (B) we obtain a value of 0.037 using the protection limit 0.60 mcGy per hr. The value of B is used to read the slant thickness (S) of the lead from figure 8-6. This yields a value of 2.5 cm for S, and the physical thickness T is 1.7 cm based on 46.2° for θ.

Problems

1. Determine the thickness of concrete needed in the floor of the brachytherapy room shown in figure 8-3 to protect personnel below the room. The distance between the floors is 14'.

2. Calculate the amount of lead needed in the door to the brachytherapy room.

9

Reports and Room Surveys

The Radiation Shielding Report

In order to be qualified to prepare shielding designs, a physicist must meet certain standards set forth by the state radiological health agency. Typically, the standards are similar to those required for certification as a health or radiological physicist by the appropriate professional board. After the planning stage for the radiation therapy facility is completed by a qualified physicist, a report of the shielding analysis is prepared and presented to the architect, owner of the facility, and the state radiological health agency. The report is forwarded to the proper state agency for review and approval. If modifications of the shielding design are required by the state, a revised report is prepared and submitted for final approval. Construction of the treatment room shielding is not initiated until final approval is granted by the state radiological health unit. A copy of the shielding report must be retained by the owner or by the person in charge of the installation. The following is a description of an acceptable shielding report for a medical accelerator facility.

Cover Page

The cover page of the report should include the following elements:

1. Title that identifies the shielding report
2. Name and address of the medical facility
3. Identification of the therapy accelerator
4. Building and room location of the accelerator
5. Name, address, title, and telephone number of the radiological physicist who prepared the report
6. Date the report was submitted to the state agency.

Introduction

The introduction should include all specific conditions that have been used for the shielding evaluation. The following are typical parameters:

1. Radiation source—manufacturer and model of accelerator, megavoltage of x-ray beams and method of specifying the megavoltage, and energy of electron beams.
2. Head leakage—value of the neutron and x-ray head leakage.
3. Workload (W)—cGy at the isocenter in seven days of operation and cGy at the isocenter in any one hour of operation of the x-ray beam.
4. Use factor (U)—typically 1/4 is used for each wall, floor, and ceiling. However, if total body irradiation is to be conducted, the workload and use factors may be different.
5. Shielding materials—list density and other shielding properties of the various materials used to construct the treatment vault.
6. Location of the HVAC penetration—typically in the wall above the treatment room door.
7. Location of conduit for physics cables.
8. Recesses in the walls—recesses made for junction boxes, etc., must be backed by steel or lead plates of a certain thickness to retain the recommended shielding value.
9. Radiation protection criteria used to analyze the shielding requirements.
10. If a beam stop is to be used, the transmission of the beam through the device should be less than 0.1% including phantom scatter up to 30° off the central axis of the beam with maximum collimator opening. The range of gantry angles over which the beam stop must be in the beam should be stated.

Include the following statements:

11. Drawings provided by the architects were assumed to represent the radiation treatment facility accurately.
12. The primary barriers will be centered on the isocenter.
13. No change of the isocenter location or additional penetrations will be made in the shielding without review by a qualified radiological physicist.
14. Before construction begins the final drawings for the facility must be reviewed by a qualified radiological physicist.

Methods of Shielding Calculations

The next section should describe methods of shielding calculation and list references as to their source (NCRP Reports, etc.). Special attention should be given to the methods used to design laminated shields, maze doors, and direct shielded doors.

Shielding Requirements

Shielding thickness values and the types of materials to be used should be tabulated and marked on drawings of the treatment facility. In addition, values of the distance (d) from the radiation source to the point protected are listed, and controlled and uncontrolled areas are identified and referenced to the floor plan for the facility. The locations of the primary and secondary barriers are indicated on the room drawings as well as the target rotational plane. The width of each primary barrier should be indicated, and separate figures may be needed to depict the door design and HVAC baffle layouts.

Facility Drawings

Drawings of the treatment room and maze scaled to 1/4" = 1' showing the position of the isocenter and the target rotational plane are included in the shielding report. Both vertical section views and plot or floor plans are included. Information about occupancy in areas adjacent to the shielding barriers should be shown on the drawings.

Construction Inspection

After the shielding design has been approved by the state radiological health unit, construction of the accelerator vault begins. An inspection by a qualified radiological physicist during construction of the facility is recommended. Some of the items that should be evaluated are listed below:

1. Thickness and density of concrete
2. Thickness of metal shielding and polyethylene used for neutron shielding
3. Shielding behind recesses in concrete (laser boxes, etc.)
4. HVAC shielding if used
5. Location of pipe for physics cables
6. Inspection to determine if required shielding design was followed

A letter outlining any items of noncompliance should be prepared by the physicist and distributed to the state agency, the owner of the facility, and the architectural firm.

Radiation Shielding Survey

Following the construction of a new installation the accelerator is installed and made operational. A preliminary survey is carried out at the time of first beam to ensure that there are no radiological health hazards to the installation engineer and personnel near the facility. Once the accelerator has been made completely operational and the initial calibration has been carried out, a complete shielding survey such as the one described below is conducted.

Survey Equipment

The equipment needed to perform the room survey includes the following items:

1. Portable ionization chamber survey instrument for photon measurements. The instrument should have both a rate and integration mode and a range from 0 to 5 R per hour.
2. Geiger-Müller counter
3. Portable neutron survey instrument
4. Scattering phantom
5. X-ray film such as Kodak XV/2 if the photon head leakage is to be evaluated. An integrating ionization chamber is used for the measurement of the photon head leakage.
6. Moderated foil activation dosimeter and associated foil counting system if the neutron head leakage is to be measured.
7. Ionization chamber to spot check the output of the accelerator.
8. Accessories: hard hat, rain gear, old clothes, plastic bags to cover instruments in case of rain, walkie-talkies, rope and backpack for hoisting instruments to the roof area, stopwatch, flashlight, etc.

Dosimeters Used for the Room Survey

A. Photons

An evaluation of the photon level outside the shielding barriers is carried out using a portable ionization chamber survey meter. The author has found that an ionization chamber pressurized to about six atmospheres will allow measurements from approximately 0.05 mR per hour to 5 R per hour. This range of exposure rates is more than adequate for most barrier surveys. The instrument response as a function of photon energy is flat to within ± 10% in the range 0.025 MeV to 1.25 MeV, and an over-response of 15% was noted for ^{16}N gamma rays (6.06 to 8.89 MeV). If the head leakage is to be measured, an analog-type instrument should be used in place of the more up-to-date digital dosimetry due to interference caused by the pulsed beam of the accelerator and microwave radiation in the accelerator room. A condenser chamber with a maximum scale reading of 0.25 R is convenient for use in head leakage measurements. This chamber has a cross-sectional area of 10 cm^2 along the major axis, which produces a reading averaged over the recommended area for head leakage evaluation. The thickness of the chamber wall is adequate for leakage radiation measurements from accelerators operating as high as 25 MeV (McGinley and Persons 1995a). A ^{137}Cs source whose activity has been established by the National Institute of Standards and Technology (NIST) is used to calibrate the survey meters employed to measure the head leakage and dose rate outside the barriers. The calibration is repeated on an annual basis, and a check source should be used quarterly to ensure that the dosimeter is operating properly.

B. Neutrons

Since most physicists are not thoroughly familiar with neutron dosimetry, a review of basic neutron physics is in order. Neutrons are classified in terms of their energy as follows.

1. Slow neutrons—energy less than 0.5 eV. Sometimes the term "thermal neutrons" is used in place of "slow neutrons." However, the expression "thermal neutrons" implies that the neutrons have a Maxwellian velocity distribution with a most probable velocity of 2,200 m s^{-1}. This velocity corresponds to an energy of 0.025 eV. The Maxwellian distribution has very few neutrons with energy greater than 0.5 eV.

2. Intermediate energy neutrons—energy range from 0.5 eV to tens of keV energy.
3. Fast neutrons—energy range from few tens of keV upward.

Neutrons deposit dose in tissue by interactions at the nuclear level with the major tissue elements (H, C, O, and N). Neutron reactions with hydrogen produce the majority of the dose delivered to tissue by neutrons of all energies. Elastic scattering of neutrons by hydrogen contributes at least 75% of the dose over the fast neutron energy range. When an elastic scattering event occurs, the hydrogen nucleus recoils as a proton. Neutron capture by hydrogen, which produces a gamma ray of 2.21 MeV energy, results in the majority of the dose delivered to tissue by slow neutrons. Next of importance for slow neutrons is the nuclear reaction with ^{14}N, which produces a 0.6 MeV proton. The reactions responsible for most of the dose produced by neutrons in tissue are outlined below.

Fast neutrons:	$^{1}H(n,n)^{1}H$	proton recoil
Slow neutrons:	$^{1}H(n,\gamma)^{2}H$	neutron capture
	$^{14}N(n,p)^{14}C$	nuclear reaction

Both elastic scattering by hydrogen and nuclear reactions with nitrogen produce charged particles that have high linear energy transfer (LET) in biological tissues. Since the majority of the dose delivered to tissue by neutrons is produced by high LET-charged particles, the quality factor (Q) associated with neutrons is in the range of 2 to 10. It has been suggested that the upper limit of the quality factor should be increased to 20 for fast neutrons. Photons, on the other hand, generate high-energy electrons in tissue that have low LET as compared with the charged particles produced by neutrons. The quality factor assigned to photons is 1, and the dose equivalent (H) and absorbed (D) are the same in size. The dose equivalent is evaluated from the dose as shown by equation 9-1.

$$H = Q\,D \tag{9-1}$$

where

H = dose equivalent (Sv)
Q = quality factor
D = absorbed dose (Gy).

The dosimetry of neutrons is complicated by the fact that the neutron energy spectrum is usually needed for an accurate evaluation of the dose equivalent. This can be seen from figure 9-1, which is a plot of the dose equivalent rate produced by unit neutron flux as a function of neutron energy. A variation of the dose equivalent rate per unit neutron flux of approximately a factor of 40 is seen over the energy range from slow to fast neutrons. Neutron fields in the treatment room and outside the shielding are composed of slow, intermediate, and fast neutrons. To eliminate the need for complex neutron spectral measurement when neutron dosimetry is carried out, the "remmeter" was developed. This device is composed of a neutron moderator with a slow neutron detector at its center. Neutrons that enter the moderator are reduced in energy by elastic collisions, and some of the low-energy neutrons produce a response in the slow neutron detector. The moderator is designed so that the response rate of the detector per unit neutron flux as a function of neutron energy has the same shape as the curve shown in figure 9-1. Calibration of the dosimeter is carried out using a neutron source with a known energy spectrum. For example, the calibration can be conducted using a ^{252}Cf neutron source housed in a heavy water moderator. The moderated fission spectrum produced by the heavy water is similar to the neutron energy spectrum outside a concrete barrier. The calibration factor established by this method is used to relate the instrument response to the neutron dose equivalent or neutron dose equivalent rate. Measurements made in a neutron field with an unknown and different energy spectrum can be converted to the neutron dose equivalent rate using the calibration factor. This feature of the dosimeter, which allows it to be used without knowledge of the neutron energy distribution, is a result of the matching of the instrument response to the curve shown in figure 9-1.

A number of remmeter moderators, some of which are listed below, have been developed for health protection work. The 10" polyethylene sphere, which is quite heavy, can be reduced in weight by employing a 9" diameter sphere that has an internal cadmium absorber located close to the slow neutron detector. Both the 10" and 9" spheres over-respond to intermediate energy neutrons, and an improved match to the curve of figure 9-1 can be obtained with the Braun-Anderson moderator, which is a cylindrical polyethylene moderator 21.6 cm in diameter and 24.4 cm long with an internal cadmium absorber. However, it has been the author's experience that the

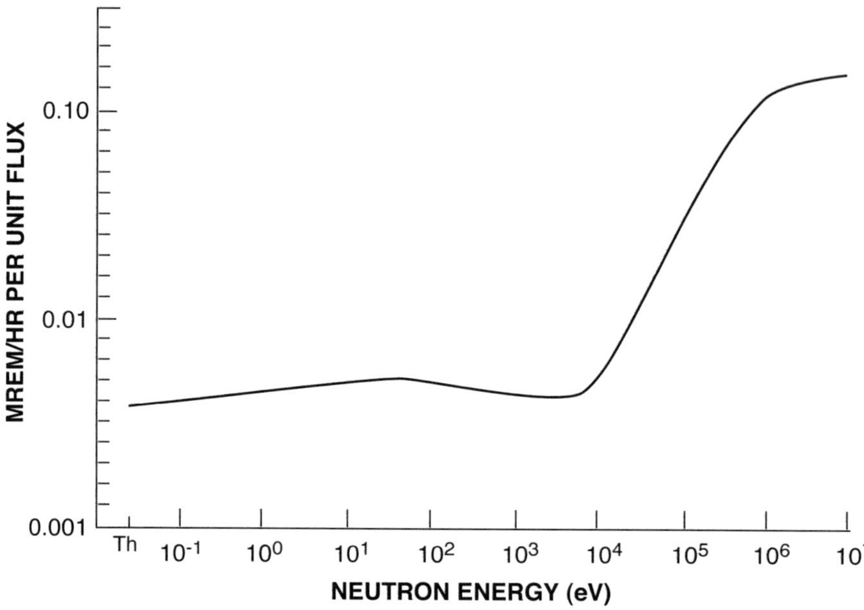

Figure 9-1. Neutron dose equivalent rate produced by unit neutron flux as a function of neutron energy. Based on data from NCRP Report No. 63 (NCRP 1957).

response of each of the dosimeters listed in Table 9-1 is similar for the neutron field that exists outside the shielding of medical accelerators.

Table 9-1 Remmeter moderators and their associated slow neutron detector

Moderator	*Slow neutron detector*
Polyethylene sphere (10" diameter)	BF_3 proportional counter
	^{6}LiI scintillation counter
	Activation foils (Au and In)
Polyethylene sphere (9" diameter with internal Cd absorber)	BF_3 proportional counter
Braun-Anderson moderator	BF_3 proportional counter

Most commercial portable survey instruments employ the BF_3 proportional counter system to detect slow neutrons at the center of the moderator. This detector relies on the neutron reaction ^{10}B (n,α)^{7}Li, which has a high cross section for thermal neutrons. The alpha particle and recoil ^{7}Li nucleus produce a large pulse in the proportional counter that can be discriminated from the small pulses produced by photons. The ^{6}LiI scintillation detector is quite sensitive to pulsed photon fields (McGinley and McCranie 1984) and should not be used for surveys at medical accelerator facilities. Measurements cannot be made in the treatment room with the portable survey instruments mentioned above due to the intense pulsed photon field produced when the accelerator is operated. Activation detectors do not suffer from interference caused by pulsed photons and can be used for neutron head leakage and patient plane measurements. Either gold or indium foils can be used in the moderator and the induced radioactivity produced by slow neutron capture in the foil measured after the irradiation. A ^{252}Cf neutron source is used to calibrate the moderated activation system in order to establish a relationship between the foil counts per unit time and the neutron dose equivalent rate.

A moderator that can be used to determine the fast neutron flux density in the treatment room has been described by Stephens and Smith (1958). This device, which is referred to as a fluxmeter, consists of an indium foil placed at the center of a 6″ diameter paraffin sphere encased in a cadium thermal neutron shield. The activity of the indium foil produced by neutron capture has been shown to be directly proportional to the neutron flux density at the point of measurement for neutrons in the energy range 20 keV to 20 MeV. The dosimetry system is calibrated by use of a ^{252}Cf source of known strength. If the energy spectrum of the neutron field is known, the neutron flux density can be converted to the dose equivalent rate due to fast neutrons. When the system is used to measure the neutron flux density in the x-ray beam, corrections are needed to account for the response produced by neutrons generated by photon interactions in the cadmium shield (McGinley and Kelly 1987).

By exposing the indium foil without the moderator and shield, an estimate of the dose equivalent rate due to slow neutrons can be made and added to the fast neutron dose equivalent rate. The determination of the slow neutron dose equivalent requires two measurements, one with the foil shielded from slow neutrons with a cadmium cover and a second using a bare foil. The response due to slow neutrons is proportional to the difference between the unshielded and shielded foil. The detector must be calibrated similarly to the other dosimeters described above in a known neutron field.

The following equation is used to correct the count rate of a foil used in one of the moderators mentioned above or for slow neutron measurements. Equation 9-2 gives the count rate $(c/s)_s$ at the end of the irradiation corrected for decay and lack of saturation.

$$(c/s)_S = \frac{\lambda(\text{total counts})e^{\lambda t_d}}{(1-e^{-\lambda t_i})(1-e^{-\lambda t_c})} \tag{9-2}$$

where

t_d = decay time (s)
t_c = counting time (s)
t_i = irradiation time (s)
λ = decay constant (s^{-1}) = 0.693/half-life.

Survey Measurements

After the accelerator has been commissioned, the shielding survey is carried out. Review the shielding plans before beginning the survey in order to spot the worst-case conditions. For your own safety realize that unreported changes in the construction of the facility can result in high dose levels outside the shielding. A GM survey instrument is used to scan the barriers for voids and cracks, and the neutron and photon survey instruments discussed above are employed to establish the dose equivalent rate outside the shielding. The accelerator is operated at maximum x-ray dose rate during the survey. Remember to check uncontrolled areas behind controlled areas.

When measuring behind primary barriers, use a maximum field size without a scattering phantom. The collimator is rotated (45°) to produce the maximum field width. Gantry angles of 0°, 90°, 180°, and 270° are used as well as a number of angles off the vertical up beam direction for tapered ceiling shields. Always check for leakage at the junction of the ceiling slab and the primary walls, especially if the primary wall is part metal and part concrete. The measurements are made at a distance of 30 cm from the barrier, and a simple distance rod attached to the survey instrument will be helpful.

The secondary barriers are surveyed in a similar fashion but with a scattering phantom in the beam. Be on the lookout for leakage produced by small angle scatter near primary barriers. The door and HVAC duct should be surveyed for neutrons and photons. This is the only area where neutrons are commonly found in an all-concrete treatment room. Measurements should be made outside the facility at a number of distances from the isocenter to determine radiation levels due to skyshine. If a tall building is located adjacent to the treatment room, the upper floors of the building should be checked for skyshine radiation and leakage from a thin ceiling slab or an atrium. The measurements are recorded along with the location and irradiation parameters.

In carrying out the survey one should be aware of the many nuisances that may be encountered, such as anxious contractors and hospital administrators, offices occupied by excitable nonradiation workers, lack of access to locked rooms and the roof area, etc. Be prepared for mud, bad weather, construction litter, and roof areas that can only be reached by a rickety ladder.

Head leakage surveys are infrequently done because state radiological agencies will accept typical data for the accelerator based on information supplied by the manufacturer. Measurement of the neutron head leakage using an activation foil system requires a calibration of the dosimetry system with a neutron source of known strength, and few calibration laboratories offer neutron calibration for a moderated activation system. A simple method for determining the neutron head leakage outside the main x-ray beam is to use bubble detectors. These devices are relatively inexpensive and are calibrated by the manufacturer in terms of the number of bubbles produced by unit dose equivalent. The device consists of super-heated droplets suspended in a gel, and the gel is contained in a vial about the size of a test tube. When neutrons interact with the gel or a droplet, recoil protons are produced that can cause the droplet to become a bubble. The number of bubbles produced are directly related to the neutron dose equivalent at the point of measurement. Bubble detectors should not be used in the main x-ray beam because photon interactions in the dosimeter will generate neutrons that will be detected by the device and result in a neutron dose equivalent that is too large.

Bubble detectors are also available that can be used to determine the head leakage component from photons. A condenser ionization chamber can also be used to evaluate the photon head leakage. These chambers are calibrated using a ^{137}Cs source of known strength. Before beginning the photon measurements, x-ray film is used to cover the head and accelerator structure of the linear accelerator. The accelerator is then operated to produce a dose on the order of 5000 cGy at the isocenter, and the film is developed. "Hot" spots can be located with this technique, and an ion chamber used to confirm the leakage level.

The Shielding Evaluation Report

The shielding evaluation report should contain the following items:

1. Title page—type of radiation unit, location, date of survey, and name of the person who performed the survey and prepared the report.
2. Methods—description of survey technique used, method of calculation of the dose equivalent in any one hour of operation, dose equivalent in seven days of operation, and annual dose equivalent. Values are given of the workload (W), occupancy factors (T), and utilization factors (U) used in the calculations.
3. Instruments used for survey—model serial number and date of calibration.
4. Results—value of maximum dose equivalent rate measured at points outside the shielding barriers, gantry angle, location, and dose rate at the isocenter. Table of the maximum dose equivalent to be expected at various points outside the shielding for any one hour, in any seven consecutive days of operation, and in one year are prepared. The table should indicate the W, U, and T values used and the type of area (controlled, uncontrolled, or restricted).
5. Conclusions and recommendations—If the shielding is acceptable, a statement indicating that the facility meets the codes and guidelines of the state radiological health agency is made and the relevant protection guidelines are quoted. If items of noncompliance are found, specific recommendations to correct the problems are given. Indication should be given if a follow-up survey is needed.
6. Floor plan and section views of the treatment facility—Survey points are correlated with the results tables, and the various areas outside the shielding are identified.

Problems

1. The room shown in figure 9-2 was designed for a 10 MeV accelerator. It has been decided to upgrade the room to house a dual energy accelerator (6 and 18 MV x-rays based on the British Journal of Radiology Supplement No. 11). Note that a multilevel building is located 60' from the treatment room.
   a. Discuss the room changes that will be needed for the upgrade.
   b. Prepare a shielding evaluation report for the upgrade.

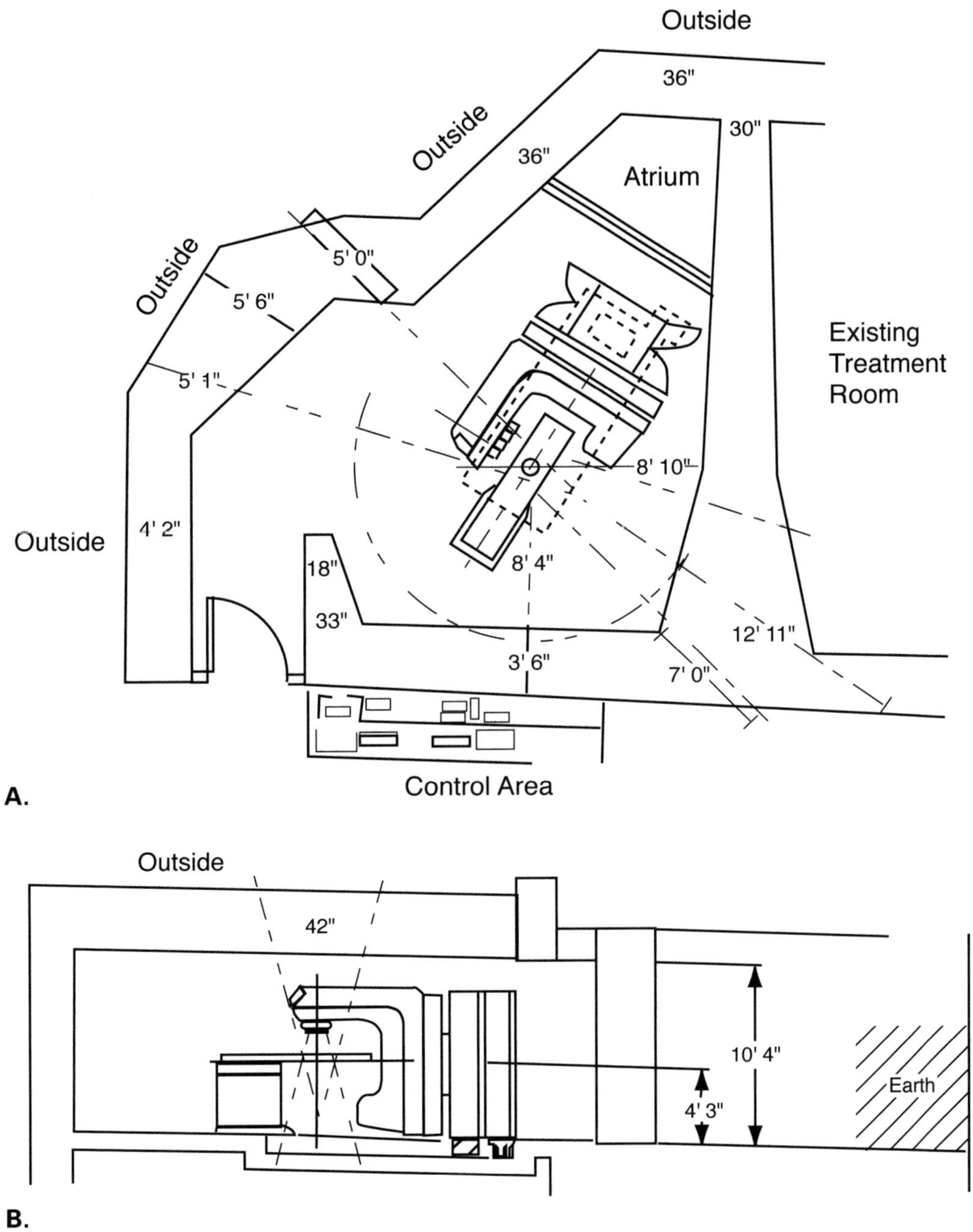

Figure 9-2. Floor plan and section view of treatment room to be upgraded for an 18 MeV accelerator A. Floor plan view, where floor is 7′6″ below grade outside. B. Section view in Gantry Plane

2. Prepare a shielding evaluation report for a new treatment room that will house a dual energy (6 and 18 MeV) medical accelerator.
3. Carry out a radiation survey at your hospital or clinic for a high-energy accelerator and turn in a shielding survey report.

References

Almen, A.; Ahlgren, L.; Mattsson, S. Absorbed dose to technicians due to induced activity in linear accelerators for radiation therapy. Phys. Med. Biol. 36:815–822; 1991.

AAPM. A protocol for the determination of absorbed dose from high energy photon and electron beams. Med. Phys. 10:741–771; 1983.

Barish, J.R. On designing room shielding for total-body irradiation. Health Phys. 70:714–716; 1996.

Berman, B.L. Atlas of photoneutron cross sections obtained with monoenergetic photons. UCRL 78482; 1976.

Biggs, P.J. Obliquity factors for ^{60}Co and 4, 10 and 18 MV x-rays for concrete, steel, and lead and angles of incidence between 0° and 70°. Health Phys. 70:527–536; 1996.

British Journal of Radiology (BJR) Supplement No. 11. Central axis depth dose data for use in radiotherapy; 1972.

British Journal of Radiology (BJR) Supplement No. 17. Central axis depth dose data for use in radiotherapy; 1983.

Fenn, J.O.; McGinley, P.H. Stray photoneutron fields produced by the GE Saturne accelerator. Radiat. Protect. Management 12:39–45; 1995.

Glasser, O. Wilhelm Conrad Roentgen and the early history of the roentgen rays. Springfield, Illinois: Charles C. Thomas Publishing Company; 1934.

Henshaw, P.S. Further problems in x-ray protection. Radiol. 44:569–580; 1945.

Kaye, G.W.C. Some fundamental aspects of roentgen rays and the protection of the roentgen-ray worker. Am. J. Roentgenol. 18:401–425; 1927.

Kersey, R.W. Estimation of neutron and gamma radiation doses in the entrance maze of SL 75-20 linear accelerator treatment rooms. Medicamundi 24:151–155; 1979.

Kerst, D.W. The acceleration of electrons by magnetic induction. Phys. Rev. 60:47–53; 1941.

Klech, J.H.; Elsalim, M. Clinical workloads and use factors for medical linear accelerators. Med. Phys. 21:952; 1994.

Kliauga, P.; Amols, H. Photoneutrons from high energy medical linear accelerators. Int. J. Rad. Oncology Biol. Phys. 31:629–633; 1995.

Lokan, K.H.; Sherman, N.K.; Gellie, W.H.; Henry, W.H.; Levesque, R.; Nowack, A.; Teather, G.G.; Lunquist, J.R. Bremsstrahlung attenuation measurements in ilmenite loaded concrete. Health Phys. 23:193–199; 1972.

Maruyama, T.; Kumamoto, Y.; Kato, Y.; Hashizume, T.; Yamamoto, M. Attenuation of 4-32 MV x-rays in ordinary concrete, heavy concrete, iron and lead. Health Phys. 20:277–284; 1971.

McCall, R.C.; Jenkins, T.M.; Shorc, R.A. Transport of acceleration produced neutrons in a concrete room. IEEE Transactions on Nuclear Science NS-26:1593–1602; 1979.

McCall, R.C. Neutron yield of medical electron accelerators, SLAC-Pub-4480, Stanford, California; 1987.

McGinley, P.H.; Wright, B.A.; Meding, C.J. Dose to radiotherapy technologist from air activation. Med. Phys. 11:855–858; 1984.

McGinley, P.H.; McCranie, E. The sensitivity of two remmeters to leakage x-rays from medical accelerators. Health Phys. 46:471–474; 1984.

McGinley, P.H.; Kelly, C.J. Photoneutron production in the cadmium thermal neutron shield of a neutron detector. Conference Proceedings of the Twentieth Midyear Topical Symposium of the Health Physics Society. Conf-8602106:244–249; February 1987.

McGinley, P.H. Photoneutron dose levels produced by the Siemens KD medical accelerator. Emory Univ. J. Med. 2:40–46; 1988.

McGinley, P.H.; Long, K.; Kaplan, R. Production of photoneutrons in a lead shield by high energy x-rays. Phys. Med. Biol. 33:975–980; 1988.

McGinley, P.H.; Landry, J.C. Neutron contamination of x-ray beams produced by the Varian Clinac 1800. Phys. Med. Biol. 34:777-783; 1989.

McGinley, P.H.; Butker, E.K. Evaluation of neutron dose equivalent at the maze entrance of medical accelerator treatment rooms. Med. Phys. 18:279–281; 1991.

McGinley, P.H. Photoneutron production in the primary barriers of medical accelerator rooms. Health Phys. 62:359–363; 1992a.

McGinley, P.H. Photoneutron fields in medical accelerator rooms with barriers constructed of concrete and metals. Health Phys. 63:698–701; 1992b.

McGinley, P.H. Design of therapy facilities. In: Eichholz, G.G.; Shonka, J.J., eds. Hospital health physics, Proceedings of the 1993 Health Physics Society Summer School. Richland, Washington: Research Enterprises Publishing: 53–67;1993a.

McGinley, P.H. Radiation skyshine produced by an 18 MeV medical accelerator. Radiat. Protect. Management 10:59–64; 1993b.

McGinley, P.H.; Ghavidel, S.; Landry, J.C. A study of photoneutron dose levels produced by the Phillips SL medical accelerators. Radiat. Protect. Management 10:45–50; 1993.

McGinley, P.H.; Butker, E. Laminated primary ceiling barriers for medical accelerator rooms. Phys. Med. Biol. 39:1331–1336; 1994.

McGinley, P.H.; Persons, T.M. Neutron and photon dose levels produced by field shaping blocks and a multileaf collimator. Radiat. Protect. Management 12:49–54; 1995a.

McGinley, P.H.; Miner, M.; Mitchum, M.L. A method for calculating the dose due to capture gamma rays in accelerator rooms. Phys. Med. Biol. 40:1467–1473; 1995b.

McGinley, P.H.; Miner, M.S. A method of eliminating the maze door of medical accelerator rooms. Radiat. Protect. Management 12:29–37; 1995c.

McGinley, P.H.; James, J.L. Dose levels in the maze of medical accelerator rooms. Midyear Topical Meeting of the Health Physics Society, Health Physics of Radiation Generating Machines. San Jose, California; 1997.

Morgan, S.; Morgan, H.M.; Lillicrap, S.C. Dose rate and energy spectrum in the maze of a linear accelerator treatment room. Brit. J. of Radiology 68:1237–1241; 1995.

Mutscheller, A. Physical standards of protection against roentgen-ray dangers. Am. J. Roentgenol. 13:65–70; 1925.

Mutscheller, A. Further studies on physical standards of protection against roentgen-ray dangers. Radiol. 6:314–319; 1926.

National Bureau of Standards. X-ray protection. NSB Handbook No. 60; 1955.

National Bureau of Standards. Protection against neutron radiation up to 30 million electron volts. NSB Handbook No. 63; 1957.

National Council on Radiation Protection and Measurements. Shielding for high-energy electron accelerator installations. Washington, DC: NCRP, NCRP Report No. 31; 1964.

National Council on Radiation Protection and Measurements. Structural shielding design and evaluation for medical use of x-ray and gamma rays of energies up to 10 MeV. Washington, DC: NCRP, NCRP Report No. 49; 1976.

National Council on Radiation Protection and Measurements. Radiation protection design guidelines for 0.1–100 MeV particle accelerator facilities. Washington, DC: NCRP, NCRP Report No. 51; 1977.

National Council on Radiation Protection and Measurements. Neutron contamination from medical accelerators. Bethesda, MD: NCRP, NCRP Report No. 79; 1984.

Nelson, W.R.; LaRiviere, P.D. Primary and leakage radiation calculations at 6, 10 and 25 MeV. Health Phys. 47:811–818; 1984.

Numark, N.J.; Kase, K.R. Radiation transmission and scattering for medical linacs producing x-rays of 6 and 15 MV. Health Phys. 48:289–295; 1985.

O'Brien, P.; Michaels, H.B.; Gillies, B.; Aldrich, J.E.; Andrew, J.W. Radiation protection aspects of a new high-energy linear accelerator. Med. Phys. 12:101–107; 1985.

Profio, E.A. Radiation shielding and dosimetry. New York: John Wiley & Sons; 1979.

Rollins, W.H. Roentgen-light notes. Elect. Rev. 33:107; 1898.

Rollins, W.H. Non-radiable cases for x-light tubes. Elect. Rev. 40:795–799; 1902.

Rollins, W.H. Notes on x-light. Boston: privately printed; 1904.

Stephens, L.D.; Smith, A.R. Fast neutron surveys using indium foil activation. U.S. AEC Rep. UCRL-8418; 1958.

Tesla, N. On reflected roentgen rays. Elect. Rev. 29:171–176; 1896.

Thomson, E. Roentgen ray burns. Am. X-Ray J. 3:451–453; 1898.

Tochlin, E.; LaRiviere, P.D. Attenuation of primary and leakage radiation in concrete for x-rays from a 10 MV linear accelerator. Health Phys. 36:387–392; 1979.

Varian 1991. Clinac and Ximatron typical shielding, data notes and tables. Palo Alto, California: Varian Corp.; 1991.

Weise, H.P.; Jost, P. Shielding against scattered radiation at electron accelerator installations. ESIS Newsletter 45:3–7; 1983.

Index